THE

POWER

OF THE BITE

Learn how to eat what you really like and lose weight too. On a daily basis, leaving behind just two bites of your deluxe fast-food cheeseburger or one-third of your bagel or a couple bites of your candy bar will result in losing around twelve pounds in a year. You only need to lose four ounces (a quarter pound) a week to accomplish this. Imagine what you can do with even fewer bites.

THE

POWER

OF THE BITE

Impressive Weight Loss,
One Bite at a Time

Michael A. Nierenberg, M.D.

Harvard Medical School Graduate
Adjunct Clinical Professor of Medicine, Emeritus
Stanford University

iUniverse, Inc.
New York Lincoln Shanghai

The Power of the Bite
Impressive Weight Loss, One Bite at a Time

iUniverse books may be ordered through booksellers or by contacting:

iUniverse
2021 Pine Lake Road, Suite 100
Lincoln, NE 68512
www.iuniverse.com
1-800-Authors (1-800-288-4677)

ISBN-13: 978-0-595-39963-5 (pbk)
ISBN-13: 978-0-595-84351-0 (ebk)
ISBN-10: 0-595-39963-0 (pbk)
ISBN-10: 0-595-84351-4 (ebk)

Printed in the United States of America

CONTENTS

PREFACE

A SIMPLE WEIGHT LOSS PROGRAM
FOR THE REST OF US

I gave a copy of the first draft of this book to my friend John Cassidy, cofounder of Klutz Books, to see if it might be publishable. He read the manuscript and wrote his take, beautifully capturing my purpose.

Do you laugh at temptation? Do your friends shake their heads while gazing at the fortress of your will? Do the words "bullet-proof" come up when they discuss your powers of restraint and self-discipline? Then I suggest you close this book and carefully put it back on the shelf, and get out of here. You don't need this book. You don't need any book. Apply your iron fist to your life and cut food intake without remorse. At the same time, devote a minimum of one hour a day to aerobic exercise. I recommend the hour before dawn, followed by a needle-shower of icy cold water. Have fun.

But …

If you are a normal member of the human race, filled with lo-cal intentions but hi-cal hors d'oeuvres, then maybe you should stick around. What follows is a plan about real weight loss for real people living in a world full of really good hot fudge sundaes. I'll assume you want to control your weight and that your willpower is detectable but far from the stuff of legend. That being the case, this book is all you need to lose weight.

—John Cassidy

I have tried to write a book for real people like myself, setting forth a guide to weight management that is straightforward and simple, an approach that works in the real world where we have more to do than simply focus on our weight. It is a plan for "the rest of us."

TRUISMS AND SEEMING CONTRADICTIONS

➢ TO LOSE WEIGHT, DON'T DIET

➢ SLOW WEIGHT LOSS IS FASTER THAN FAST WEIGHT LOSS

➢ CHANGE LITTLE THINGS TO CHANGE A LOT

➢ ONE HUNDRED CALORIES A DAY EQUALS TEN POUNDS A YEAR

➢ EAT MORE TO EAT LESS

➢ EXERCISE LESS TO EXERCISE MORE

➢ COOK MORE TO COOK LESS

➢ THE FREEZER IS YOUR FRIEND; RESTAURANTS ARE NOT

Between the first and last pages of this book you will come to understand these statements, simplify your weight loss program, and be happy to learn that weight loss is not such an intimidating undertaking after all.

WHY ANOTHER DIET BOOK?

Because *this is not really a diet book. Diets fail.* This has been proven over and over again. The diet industry generates $40 billion a year[1], yet obesity is on the rise. Since diets fail, it is obvious that the hundreds of books and articles written on dieting are not effective. So, rather than a diet book, this is a self-help book that will show you how you can take control of your eating and your weight. You will learn to lose weight easily, effectively, and permanently without suffering the agonies of dieting compounded by the agony of dieting defeat. I offer you the chance to understand weight loss and the problems surrounding it. Moreover, I offer you simple manageable solutions that are easily within your reach once you understand and become a believer in the power of one hundred and twenty tiny calories, and just a quarter pound weight loss a week. These seem like insignificant numbers, but the results will amaze you.

Why you?

If you are reading this book, it probably means you are interested in losing weight. I venture to say that you have tried to lose weight before … and failed. If this is true, I offer you the solution to successful weight loss, a solution that actually resides within yourself.

Losing weight is difficult for most people, and I can show you how to make it less so. Most diets require a level of commitment and energy that we simply do not want to give. We are busy doing things other than dieting, and frankly, we like to eat. *I can help you manage your weight subliminally. No weighing food. No long lists of do's and don'ts. No buying special foods or supplements. No meetings. No dietitians. No drastic dietary changes.*

Again, this is not a book about dieting. *The theme of this book is to simplify the weight loss process. This is a book about sustained weight loss based on life-style changes that are within the grasp of all of us … even those who have failed to lose weight before.*

Losing weight is like a magic act. At first it seems impossible, but once you know the trick, it's easy. This is a book about learning the little tricks of weight loss. I know there are many weight loss books and an equal number of approaches to losing those extra pounds. Most plans put forth complex principles and regimens. To justify their being published in the first place, they must be different and sensational. What makes this book unique is that it focuses on just a few general principles that are easy to understand and follow. It relies on small, simple, and easily manageable dietary changes with little impact on daily life, but with profound results over time. It works on nickels and dimes, not dollars. It looks for loose change under sofa cushions. Note the power of the quarter pound.

If you lose only a quarter pound (four ounces) a week, you will weigh almost twenty-five pounds less in two years. This is accomplished by cutting out only one hundred and twenty calories a day, just a few bites of food.

A successful weight loss program can actually be simple and painless. In fact, it needs to be if any of us are going to follow such a plan. Let's face it, very few of us like to give up our fun foods and pound away (forgive the pun) on a treadmill in an effort to lose weight.

This book will dispense with diets and dieting. I want to heighten your awareness of how to lose weight, and remove the dark cloud of "dieting" from over your head. Dealing with a diet every day is oppressive. Diets make you feel guilty if you fail to follow one or more of the plan's principles. A better approach is to lose weight without guilt or dark clouds. This approach is based on simple facts and principles, and it will minimally affect your life, yet lead to sustained weight loss over time. When you have lost your desired weight, the basic principles will become part of your daily life. You will not spend every day dieting or thinking about a diet. You will learn how to eat, not diet.

Why me?

Why did I write this book and why should you read it?

My training was at both Harvard and Stanford medical schools, and I remain a clinical professor on the voluntary medical faculty at Stanford. I retired from a successful internal medicine practice in Palo Alto after almost thirty years to pursue teaching and writing. I have been interested in weight management as a solution to multiple medical problems for a long time. I realized, however, that the time I spent with my patients on weight and diet would influence only those people in my practice. I wanted to help millions of people realize the goal of improving their health. This book is an attempt to reach as many of you as possible.

Working with patients for so many years, I came to realize that people, even intelligent people, do not understand weight loss.

"Doctor, I don't eat anything, and yet I can't lose weight." Diplomatically, I try to explain this is impossible. You just can't gain weight without eating. However, you can gain weight by eating more than your body needs.

"But, doctor, I eat less than so-and-so and they are not overweight." Sometimes life is unfair. Don't take it personally or as a failure. Everyone's food needs are different based on all sorts of factors.

The key for any one individual is to simply eat less and exercise more. But how much less or more? I will not ask you to look at a chart to decide how few calories a day you must eat to lose weight. The charts are generalizations; you are an individual. The charts are frustrating. They are averages. You are a person, not an average. The generalized numbers given in tables or charts must be adjusted for many things including your level of exercise, metabolic rate, etc. Usually, the number of calories a day is too low for comfort or too high to promote weight loss in any individual case. The factors that determine your specific weight loss program are just too complex to be classified on a chart of generalities. If you eat less than you do now, you will lose weight.

You can lose weight eating a whopping thirty-five hundred calories a day—if you are now eating four thousand calories a day! Simply eating less takes everything into consideration, such as how long you sleep, how much you exercise, how much you drink, and what your metabolic rate is. *It is easier to subtract the calories you do not need than to decide on the ones you do.* This method of calorie counting results in an easy, yet successful approach to a complex metabolic issue.

This book describes a simple approach to a complex problem and is meant to be practical, not theoretical, and to simplify, not mystify. Weight loss for most of us is more desire than commitment. After thirty years of watching patients succeed or fail at weight loss, I realize the need to keep this book short and sweet. The approach to weight loss is simple and easy. I have tried very hard to make the book informative, interesting, and a fast read. I have provided brief summaries at the beginning of chapters so those of you in a real hurry have the "skimming" already done for you. I will present weight loss principles so they make sense and are easy to remember and apply. The underlying principle is simple—eat less and exercise more. I focus on the manner in which you do this. I have set forth what I feel is a different and easy way to accomplish the goal of weight loss one bite at a time. I give you *the power of the quarter pound.*

Weight loss is simple, yet complex. One can eat thirty-five hundred calories a day and lose weight, or gain weight. One can eat cake, candy, and ice cream and lose weight, or gain weight. How? Read on. I make this complex question simple and easy to understand.

CHAPTER 1

LEARN HOW TO EAT, NOT HOW TO DIET

This chapter sets the stage to understand why diets don't work and helps you understand how and why this weight loss program will succeed. Interesting facts and figures are presented that show the importance of weight control. You will soon realize that the goal is to learn how to eat, not how to diet. I think this chapter is worth reading, but if you're in a hurry to get started, you can skip to Chapters 2 and 3 then come back to this one later.

The obesity crisis.

Obesity is increasing as a major national health problem, right up there with smoking. "In the United States, obesity results in an estimated 325,000 deaths annually...."[2] In 1995, obesity-related medical costs in the United States accounted for 5.7 percent of total U.S. medical expenses. That translates to over $51 billion.[3] In 2003, Ann Wolf of the University of Virginia Medical School estimated the costs to be $96.7 billion.[4] Approximately nineteen percent of the U.S. population is overweight by the age of eleven[5], and 64.5 percent of adults—about 127 million people—are overweight or obese.[6] *Obesity is not just about pants or dress size. Being overweight directly affects your health, contributing to diabetes, arthritis, high blood pressure, heart disease, stroke, and early death.* In addition, bank accounts of the overweight are reduced from medical costs related to diabetes, heart disease, high blood pressure, strokes, and arthritis. Obesity even increases the costs of seemingly unrelated diseases such as colon cancer, uterine cancer, breast cancer, kidney cancer, and gallstones. Professor John F. Banzhaf III of George Washington University Law School states that each obese person averages about $1,500 a year in additional health care costs.[7]

1

This affects not only your wallet, but also health insurance premiums. Have you noticed that all health insurance applications require a disclosure of your weight, even if they require little else?

Obesity affects all aspects of our lives, even in ways we do not realize. As an example, weight even impacts airline profitability. An article in *Popular Science*, February 2005, makes an interesting point. The average weight of passengers is increasing. If the average weight of passengers in 2000 were that of a passenger in 1991, airlines would save 350 million gallons of fuel. The cost savings to financially strapped airlines would be $275,000,000![8] And, how about fuel for cars? Think of the automobile gasoline that could be saved at $3 a gallon, affecting everything from the consequences of auto emissions to the cost of products shipped by truck.

Moral: That extra chocolate chip cookie can be costly. But so is dieting. An article from *Forbes* posted on *MSN Money* 4/12/05, lists the costs of the top ten diet plans including Jenny Craig, Weight Watchers, South Beach Diet, NutriSystem, Zone Diet, Slim-Fast, and Atkins. These diets range from being 26 percent to 152.8 percent costlier than eating regular food with no diet plan.[9] And to make matters worse, diets do not work.

Moral: You need to learn how to eat, not how to diet. The diet industry generates more than $40 billion in sales each year[10], yet we are getting heavier and heavier. This is certainly proof that diets do not work. From practical experience, you know diets over time don't work. There may be a brief period of success, but the pounds inevitably creep back. Numerous scientific studies confirm this.

One recent article in the *Journal of the American Medical Association* looked at numerous diets and confirmed that they had only limited efficacy.[11] An article in the *New England Journal of Medicine* explained that even diet pills required lifestyle modification to be effective.[12]

So, if you diet, you are likely destined to fail, but you are not alone. Don't blame yourself and feel like a failure. Don't despair. You can lose weight once you know how. Once you learn how to eat, not how to diet.

Diets work against you.

Structured diets require time and effort. Special foods must be purchased and prepared, and some plans require weighing or careful measuring. Other programs require meetings or counseling. All this adds time and expense.

Dieting is boring. Usually there are many do's and don'ts that ruin the pleasurable experience of eating. There is the "no white food rule." No pasta. No potatoes. No bread. No rice. No fun! There is the "high protein intake rule." Lots of meat, eggs, and cheese. Sounds like fun, but gets very boring. It also results in feeling poorly due to the high concentration of protein breakdown products in the blood stream, one of which is ammonia. Is it pleasant smelling ammonia? Picture it in your blood stream. In time, people just do not stay on restrictive or fad diets.

Diets ask you to expend time and effort, spend money, and give up your favorite foods so that you will ultimately fail. No wonder you can't lose weight dieting.

Society works against you.

An important part of our society is eating. Being sociable means eating. *Eating is part of living. Dieting is not.*

- ♥ Friends often go out to dinner for entertainment.
- ♥ Dining out is a way of rewarding the cook of the family for the effort needed to prepare meals during the week.
- ♥ Welcoming someone into your home usually means offering him or her something to eat.
- ♥ For many people, cooking sumptuous meals is a hobby, which of course entails eating the food that is prepared. Gourmet clubs, progressive dinners, and potlucks are everywhere.
- ♥ Everyone loves the large inexpensive buffets in Las Vegas.
- ♥ A meal is not a meal without the all-important and caloric dessert.

(Note that the candy industry does well even in financially tough times when people give up other things, but not sweets.)

You need a way to be part of this society and still lose weight. You want to go out with friends without bringing your "shake" to dinner. You want to be able to eat at friends' homes without being a nuisance. You want dessert. You want to fit in and still be fit. Dieting will not help you do this. What you will learn in the next few chapters will.

The food industry works against you.

The food industry's purpose is to sell food. The more you eat, the more they sell. Their goal is to make food appealing, which often means ramping up the fat, sugar, and salt. Food packaging is deceptive. Some items are made bite-sized to give the impression they are less caloric, though the tendency is simply to eat more of these small goodies. Labels showing calories are often deceptive and tempt us to eat what might otherwise be shunned as too caloric. For example, a label on one brand of blueberry muffins lists two hundred calories per serving. These are nice, big juicy looking muffins. And, gloriously they are only two hundred calories. How can that be? Read on. Each muffin is listed as two servings. So in fact, the two hundred calories is for half a muffin; a whole muffin is four hundred calories. Who eats half a muffin when they are packaged as whole muffins? Probably the same person who can eat one peanut or one potato chip.

The food industry also follows the fads. Look at all the low-carb items offered because of the trend of high protein diets. Low-fat items also abound. Even raisins are promoted as being fat-free, when that's the way nature makes them. *The trend toward increasing obesity started with the promotion of low-fat foods that were seen by consumers as healthy.* People simply thought they could eat more of these foods because they were low in fat. And they did, and gained weight because they were consuming more calories of lower fat food. So, we as a nation got heavier. Calories are calories. Less fat may be better for your heart, but your waistline only looks at total calories—whether from fat, protein, or carbohydrates. You can forget the hype that certain calories burn off faster than others.

You work against you.

You are trying too hard to diet. You are obsessed with losing weight. Can't eat this, can't eat that. You weigh yourself daily, or more.

Thinking about dieting and your weight all the time is oppressive. You always seem to be failing and falling short of your goal. You yield to temptation and then hate yourself. You are so careful for a while until finally you can't stand it anymore and binge on your favorite goodies. Your weight pops back on and you now have to start all over again, only to repeat the cycle. And if you aren't having enough trouble on your own, your friends are there to insist that you try some goodie or another, and the food industry is busy cooking up tempting new treats like cute little bite-sized cookies and candy bar ice creams.

Lighten up (literally and figuratively). You need a new approach to weight loss. Not a new diet or a new way of eating or living. You need to understand a few simple principles to succeed in losing weight. You will not have to focus on a rigid diet all the time. You can be happy and lighter at the same time. In the pages that follow, I give you the four-ounce diet—the four-ounce weight loss program as I prefer to call it—as salvation for those of us who have failed so many times before. Help yourself to weight loss one bite at a time.

Dieting is difficult. Weight loss is easier.

"Scott, you have high blood pressure and diabetes. You need to lose weight or you are going to have more and more medical problems."

"I know, Doctor Nierenberg, but I have tried all sorts of diets and never successfully lost weight. I know I need to lose twenty-five pounds, but I simply can't do it."

"I think you can. All I ask is that you cut your food intake just enough to lose a quarter pound a week. No diet per se. You don't need to change what you're eating, you only need to eat slightly less of it. Just find a hundred and twenty calories a day to discard. That's half a bagel."

"Doc, that's a snap. Give me something worth working toward."

"No, Scott, that's all I'm going to ask. I'm glad you agree that you can lose four ounces by next week. That means in four weeks you'll weigh a pound less."

"Doc, no problem."

"So, Scott, when I see you in a year you'll weigh twelve pounds less, and twenty-five pounds less in two years."

"Well, Doc, I don't know. Twenty-five pounds is a lot of weight to lose."

"Scott, I'm not asking for twenty-five pounds, I'm only asking for the four ounces you said you could deliver."

I've had this conversation hundreds of times during my practice. This illustrates the principle of small repeated goals adding up to a significant change. Look far ahead, but move a step at a time. Weight is gained in ounces not pounds, and it is lost that way if you are to succeed. One hundred and twenty calories a day is twelve pounds a year gained or lost. That means giving up two bites of a candy bar or one slice of bread and butter on a daily basis will lighten your load twelve pounds in a year and twenty-four pounds in two years. And that's without even including any exercise.

My mission. Your mission.

My mission is to write a short understandable book on how to lose weight simply and successfully. The approach is to be effective, yet painless. It is to be successful, yet enjoyable. It is to be guilt free. My hope is that this book will help stem the rising tide of obesity.

Your mission is simply to learn how to eat, not how to diet. You simply need to have enough interest in losing weight that you are willing to find a hundred and twenty tiny calories of food a day that you are willing to give up. Since calories are calories, you can even do this by giving up food items that you don't really like anyway—a freebee!

I would be thrilled with more than a hundred and twenty calories, and you may be willing to give up more in time. For now, we'll start with our weekly four-ounce goal yielding twelve pounds a year, pounds that will stay off. There will be no criticisms. Any weight loss is good. If you can only muster a hundred calories a day, fine. That will be ten pounds a year. Even only twenty-five calories a day (the equivalent of half a bite of your chocolate candy bar) will yield you two and a half pounds. We'll work through this together in the following chapters. On the other hand, if you are not willing to part with any calories, even the ones in foods you don't really enjoy, this book is not for you.

CHAPTER 2

THE POWER OF SMALL
IS HUGE

Summary:

This chapter puts forth the few simple principles behind this weight loss program, and illustrates the power of small steps repeated frequently. Included is how to use calories for weight loss even though you can't see calories or even understand what they are. You will learn how to lose weight without reading charts and tables about daily caloric intake. You will learn the "year-pound" concept, whereby you can easily calculate whether a food item is worth eating. Is it really "to die for," figuratively and literally? And, what is a fourteen-pound cola can?

The power of small is huge.

Forgive the pun, but let's leave the food on the table for now and talk more generally about why small is huge. ***Repeating small events adds up to significant changes over time.*** Here is a perfect example. As you know, quite often during financial transactions, fractions of a penny result from the computations. These then seem to disappear as cents are rounded up or down.

Years ago, a bank employee took advantage of this process. He wrote a program that swept the penny fractions into an account he established under a fictitious name. Millions and millions of transactions resulted in his gaining fractions of a penny repeatedly. By the time he was caught, he had made millions of dollars illustrating the power of recurring small events. How about a legal way of illustrating how small amounts of money can reap large gains? Let's say that starting at the birth of your grandchild you set up a trust fund that would put a mere dollar a day into an account for the child as long as he or she is alive. Conservatively, the account yields only three percent interest compounded only monthly. By the time your grandchild is eligible for social security at sixty-five, there will be $73,324.04 in that bank account.

Another example. People say they do not have time to exercise. What if you just walked around a typical high school track once a day? In a year, you would have walked ninety miles! That's three and a half marathons. And, you sleepyheads who like to spend more than the recommended eight hours a day sleeping, here is what each extra fifteen minutes costs you in terms of enjoying the activities of life (other than sleeping). Each week costs you one hundred and five minutes, a bit more than an hour and a half. In a month, you would lose over six hours, and more than seventy-two hours will be lost in a year. That's three days. Sleep half an hour extra per day and you lose almost a week a year. At one hour extra a day, you just slept through your two-week vacation.

So, what about weight since that is what we are supposed to be talking about? Let's say your goal is to lose ten pounds. You lose only two pounds after dieting for two months by giving up all sorts of things, and then binging on them because you were too aggressive in cutting them out in the first place. Focusing on the need to lose ten pounds as quickly as possible makes your weight loss program seem daunting.

"Will I ever get this weight off?" you ask yourself. "Not at this rate. So I might as well give up, relax, and have that piece of apple pie … and make it à la mode."

If your goal instead were to lose four ounces (a quarter pound) a week, you would lose the same two pounds in two months, and be right on target—satis-fied and happy. In under a year (ten months to be exact), you will lose your ten pounds effortlessly and keep them off. You will get to your goal by repeating small losses over and over again by giving up a few calories on a regular basis, and still eating the foods you like. You only need to cut down one hundred and twenty calories a day to lose the four ounces. One hundred and twenty calories is only a little more than one-third of a bagel, two bites of a candy bar, or a couple bites of a deluxe fast-food cheeseburger. My guess is that it would not take you much more effort to double this and lose twenty pounds in the same ten months or lose the ten pounds in five months, and keep them off.

The key is managing expectations, setting attainable goals, and achieving them … repeatedly. In fact, both people above are at the same point; it's just how they got there and how they view the process and their success. Is the glass half empty, or half full? Remember, you will never gain weight if you don't gain weight! What do I mean? No matter how gradual your weight loss, over time you will be lighter as long as you don't gain any weight back. In time you will reach your goal, it's only a question of how quickly. Weight fluctuation because of sporadic eating and an overly aggressive diet gets you nowhere except disappointed and frustrated.

Being steady and patient is the key, reminding me of the old adage "slow and steady wins the race." And slow isn't as slow as you think when you do the math. That's ten pounds a year by giving up only one hundred calories a day. This is without any exercise, which can promote even faster weight loss. Later I will show how exercise can also be almost subliminal, just like discarding only a few calories a day.

So, let's begin our journey to find easily attainable and sustainable weight loss.

Calorie counting—there really is no free lunch.

When it comes to weight loss, there may be good food, but there are no good calories. Every calorie counts. Remember one hundred extra calories a day is ten pounds a year. Even only ten extra calories a day is a pound a year. Just one daily bite of an average candy bar is almost six pounds a year. It will take you six months to work off those few extra bites of candy a year from now.

Despite what some diets suggest, you cannot "eat all you want" and still lose weight. Weight loss obeys the laws of physics. The fewer calories you take in, the less weight you will gain. The more calories you burn (through exercise), the less you will weigh. That's it. Even the fad, low carbohydrate diets when analyzed, simply result in a lower caloric intake over time.

Once again, there may be good foods, but not good calories. Certainly an apple is healthier than a cookie. But, if instead of two chocolate chip cookies, which would satisfy your dessert craving for as little as ninety-six calories, you were to eat two large apples in the course of an evening, you could consume as much as two hundred and thirty calories. You may feel more virtuous eating the apples, but realize that on a daily basis the apples represent almost twenty-five pounds of "apple weight" a year. I am not suggesting you eat cookies instead of fruit, or avoid apples. Certainly in terms of fat content and heart disease, fruit is a better choice. But when considering weight, too much of a good thing can be a bad thing. Every calorie counts, even calories from healthy foods.

I would ask you to keep in your mind that eating an extra one hundred calories a day results in a ten-pound weight gain in a year. One hundred calories is one pancake (without syrup), one light beer, one glass of wine, half a scone, two bites of a candy bar. Your job will be to find one hundred (or more) calories each day that you are willing to give up: a few bites of a cheeseburger, one less glass of wine, a couple fewer bites of candy. The more you give up each day, the more you will lose. We've set an initial goal of a quarter pound a week, so we need to find one hundred and twenty calories a day to meet this goal. The key, however, is not to give up just any one hundred and twenty calories, but rather to give up the calories in such a way that you really do not notice them or mind parting with them. You might begin by giving up foods you don't particularly care for anyway. After that, move on to dealing with your favorites. Notice, I suggested that you give up a few bites of your burger or candy bar. Would I be happy if you gave either up entirely? Yes, but you wouldn't. This would lead to unhappiness, frustration, and ultimate failure. By giving up only a small portion of your comfort foods, you will be willing to do this over a prolonged period or even a lifetime. This will result in weight loss and success over time, not just for a few weeks or months.

Let me give you some examples. Suppose you have a sandwich each day for lunch. If you simply took off the top piece of bread and flipped the two halves together to make a double-decker, you would still have a great sandwich, but save eighty plus calories a day. If you ate a sandwich every day this would add up to at least eight pounds in a year, four pounds if you had only four sandwiches a week. Notice, I did not even ask you to leave off the cheese or the mayonnaise. Again, this is to be painless. But, if you were willing to "lose the cheese," you would save another one hundred calories. And if you would "hold the mayo," another one hundred calories for a total savings of two hundred and eighty calories, which is twenty-eight pounds in a year of daily sandwiches. Go lift five standard bags of flour; that's only twenty-five pounds.

Okay, so you are not a sandwich person. You are into salads. I will deal with salads in more detail later, but for now let's just look at the dressing. I do not like diet dressings, but regular dressings can be high in calories. Here is a simple and quick solution. Buy a salad dressing that has a layer of oil at the top such as Italian, Caesar, etc. Bring it home, pour off the oil, and replace it with balsamic vinegar, which has many fewer calories than oil. (I suggest balsamic because it is less bitter than regular vinegar and enhances rather than detracts from the taste.) One quick shake and you just saved between one thousand and fifteen hundred calories per bottle. That's at least ten days' worth of your one hundred and twenty calories with no effort. Now the salads are really helping with your weight loss.

There are little calories to trim off everywhere. And the beauty is that the little ones are the easy ones to give up. They won't be missed, but they count. Save those nickels and dimes and soon you'll have a dollar, or more.

Make it a game to see how many little calories you can give up and still be very happy. Your reward will be success.

I promised you weight loss by eating candy. That is, assuming you are already eating candy rather than adding sweets to your diet. What exactly do I mean when I say you can lose weight and still eat candy?

Let's say you eat one small bag of little candy coated chocolate treats a day. Say each piece is slightly less than five calories. I would ask that when you buy the bag you open it up and immediately throw away five or six little pieces (only about ten percent of the bag). This simple act means you are giving up about twenty-five calories a day; two and a half pounds or so a year. More pieces discarded, more weight loss. I doubt you will miss the five little pieces, but your weight will. If you're unable to waste food, which you may have to rethink, you can save the five pieces for nine days and have one reduced size bag to consume as is. I caution you, however, that the stray pieces you set aside may call out to you before the nine days are up!

I want to stress that I am not condoning eating candy as a weight loss supplement. Rather, if you are already eating candy, and wish to continue doing so, moderation is the key. You can still have your candy, but just a bit less. And, if you eat it slowly like you should, you may enjoy it even more than wolfing it down while sitting in your car during rush hour.

What about another favorite like apple pie? Let's say you go to a restaurant and decide to have dessert. (I'll deal with restaurants later in more detail.) You order apple pie. When the pie comes, it is à la mode. You wanted the pie and were willing to deal with the calories, but had not counted on it being à la mode. An ethical dilemma; what to do? A happy solution is to push the ice cream aside, but enjoy the pie to the fullest. This would most likely save you one hundred and fifty to two hundred calories. On a daily basis, that's fifteen to twenty pounds a year.

If you have to eat a hot fudge sundae, could you leave off the cherry? How about leaving the fruit garnish in your mai tai—that is, if you insist on having a mai tai in the first place. Again, I am not anti-fruit. We're just looking for those easy calories to discard. (I will write more about alcohol in a later chapter.)

Every bite counts.

A good approach to food is to remember that every bite counts. Given this fact, when you are eating something, be sure it is worth the calories. *When someone describes a wildly rich dessert as "to die for," you need to decide, "Is it really?"* When you are eating the dessert, is it so good that you are willing to give up other foods to compensate? Is it so good that it's worth eating even if eating it would make you gain weight and subject you to medical illnesses such as diabetes, heat attacks, and strokes? Is it truly "to die for" in the literal sense? Homemade fudge maybe; a stale candy bar left over from Halloween, I doubt it. If something were to die for, would you be willing to eat only part of it? And do only half the damage. In short, is a food worth eating in terms of the calories? If so, how much should you eat? This needs to become a subconscious thought process.

How you approach this thought process of deciding what to eat is very important. Weight management is an emotional issue for most people. Eating is fun. It is a social activity. Eating is often a reward for things well done. It is soothing when things go wrong. So then, how do you give up dessert, or cheese, or alcohol, or bread? *The key is not to give up the foods you like, but rather to eat them intelligently. Eat fewer calories and receive more satisfaction.*

Let's say you are at a cocktail party. The wine is in a box and the cheese and crackers look like they came out of your child's lunch box snack pack. Let's say you succumb to your basic instincts and eat even modestly; perhaps four crackers and cheese, and two glasses of wine. This represents five hundred to six hundred calories of unappealing food. If you were to exercise by walking, it would take you two and a half to three hours to work off these calories. If, at the cocktail party, you settle for a mineral water and some crudités, the damage would be minimal, and the satisfaction no worse based on the quality of the food. In fact, the satisfaction might be better in that you haven't eaten bad food or gained weight. I suggest that, if you want to, you go home after eating modest fare and have just one glass of good wine and the same four crackers, but with good cheese. This would taste better and save you one hundred calories to boot. Pamper yourself with better food and beverage and still lose weight.

Take note that at no point have I insisted you give up your favorites. Instead, you can start by weeding out the foods that are low on your list. Next, simply eat less of your favorites, remembering you have to deal with any calories you eat. Unfortunately, in terms of your favorites, taste appeal and high calories are often linked. In other words, I assume your favorites are not raw vegetables and mineral water. In time some of your favorite goodies may become less appealing when you consider the calories. And you certainly won't waste calories on bad food.

Consciously assessing what you eat will result in eating fewer calories and subsequent weight loss. Be sure what you eat is worth it. It is all about choice and about not feeling deprived while you make these choices. Weight loss has to be a positive experience or you cannot sustain it. There are really no "don't eat" foods, but you must be aware of what you are eating in terms of calories and the consequences. This is not a bad thing; it is a reality.

One other point I would like to make is that *different days have different do's and don'ts. A correct decision on one day may be an incorrect decision on another.* You need to consider food intake not just on a meal basis, but also on a daily and weekly basis. Is a double cheeseburger good or bad? That depends.

On a day when you eat from a breakfast buffet, have ribs and fries for lunch, the burger at dinner adds insult to injury … it's terrible. If you had oatmeal for breakfast and soup for lunch, the burger at dinner is at worst bad, but may be good if it is your treat for the week and makes you content to stay on your weight loss program. The total calories for the day are quite manageable because of your careful breakfast and lunch intake. So, it's not that any single food per se is bad; it is that the food has to be considered in the context of the rest of the day, and the rest of the week. If you are on target for the four ounces per week, let the burger slide if it makes you happy. If you are not on target, consider passing it up. Again, remember we are talking about weight, not heart-healthy foods, which a double cheeseburger will never be!

Who has ever seen a calorie? Have you ever tasted one?

So far, I have talked about cutting calories to lose weight. I have done this because everyone else talks about calories. Thinking in terms of calories can be treacherous because, as noted earlier, small numbers add up to big gains. Compared to the one hundred and eighty to four hundred calories in a blueberry muffin, the one hundred calories in an apple may seem insignificant. An apple a day keeps the doctor away because of some vitamin C and other nutrients, but over a year that apple a day will put ten pounds on your waistline! So, while the world deals in calories, we need a better concept to guide our weight loss. We need a way to picture the effect of repeatedly eating (or not eating) small numbers of calories.

What exactly is a calorie anyway?

A calorie is simply the quantity of energy required to raise one gram of water 1°C at 15°C. Now the physicists among us know what this means. But what about the rest of us? Can we see a calorie? Can we taste one? Seems like a hard concept to visualize. So, why do we always talk about calories? For one thing, everyone else does. Even if we can't picture a calorie, it is a way of comparing how much weight we gain from various foods. Calorie content enables us to know that an apple will put on less weight than a piece of apple pie, so I will often allude to calories in various foods to show the effect of eating them. The caloric values of foods are easy to obtain, and the labels on foods include calorie content. I feel a more useful way to think about food is in terms of what I call *year-pounds*. *A year-pound is the measure of what you would gain eating an item every day for a year, over and above what you normally eat.*

As an example, what is the effect on your weight if you decide to eat an extra piece of bread each day at eighty calories per slice? In a year, you would weigh eight pounds more from these bread slices, so a single slice of bread is eight *year-pounds*. Two slices of bread are sixteen *year-pounds*. Picture holding three, five-pound bags of flour, that's only fifteen pounds. Now you can appreciate the consequence of eating two pieces of bread a day above what you normally eat. To me, this concept is easier to picture and use than the calorie, an item you will never be able to see, taste, or probably understand. Let me explore this a bit more in the next section.

Year-pounds: The fourteen-pound cola can and the twenty-eight pound candy bar.

Here are a few examples of how thinking in terms of *year-pounds* will make food choices easier. Remember, choices that save calories result in weight loss.

Pick up a can of a non-diet cola. Look at the label. Calories: 140. That doesn't seem too bad. After all, you may be eating thousands of calories a day. On a daily basis, however, that cola equals fourteen pounds of calories over a year.

So when you pick up that can of cola, don't think of it as twelve ounces or one hundred and forty calories, think of it as fourteen year-pounds. Fourteen pounds is almost three, five-pound bags of sugar. Try lifting that. Thinking of the canned cola this way, you may opt for water, iced tea, or a diet drink. *Think of a loaded cheeseburger at a fast food restaurant (the burger can run five hundred calories or more), not as five hundred calories, but as fifty year-pounds.*

And how about that twenty-eight pound candy bar? A plain milk chocolate bar is about one hundred and forty-eight calories per ounce. On a daily basis, one candy bar a day is about twenty-three pounds a year. Chocolate candy bars with other ingredients may run a little less per ounce, but since they tend to be larger, the total calories are more like two hundred and eighty each. So, your candy bar weighs in at twenty-eight *year-pounds*, or about five and a half *year-pounds* per bite. Are you really sure you want it? Maybe not. But if you are, eat it and enjoy it, but be aware of the consequences. Don't feel guilty or beat yourself up. You made an intelligent decision at the time. Life and food are to be enjoyed. Remember, no absolute "don'ts" in my approach—only intelligent, informed choices.

Okay. You get the idea of the *year-pound*, but who has the time to figure it out for various foods? It is really very simple and fast. Look at a label. Find the calories per serving (more about reading labels later). Divide this number by ten. The result is the number of *year-pounds* per serving. What could be easier? Two hundred and fifty calories, twenty-five *year-pounds*. Three hundred calories, thirty *year-pounds*. Even a number like 272 calories is easy. Move the decimal one place to the left and you get 27.2 *year-pounds*. Thinking of food in this way makes more sense than calories. *You can't imagine fifty calories, but you know what five pounds feels like.*

Food that really *is* to die for.

Thinking in terms of *year-pounds*, you may be inclined to avoid everything because every calorie counts, and on a yearly basis even an apple gets a value of ten *year-pounds*. Don't develop an eating phobia. Do remember that you need to eat. For instance, an average diet needed to maintain weight and health might be around fifteen hundred to twenty-five hundred calories. I am not aiming to make you afraid of food, but rather getting you to make choices within your daily calories to maximize both your enjoyment and your weight loss. Hence, the concept *"to die for"* can be a positive as well as a negative.

What I am saying is you need to eat, and there really is food "to die for." You do not need to give up your favorite foods even if they are high calorie items like pecan pie and French fries. You simply have to eat less of them and deal with the calories you do eat. Consciously assessing what you frequently eat will result in fewer calories and promote subsequent weight loss. Being sure that what you eat is worth it will enhance what you're eating. No stuffing on stale potato chips. If you're going to eat chips, realize the consequences, so at least insist on fresh ones.

How about that prepackaged cinnamon roll and the mediocre coffee from the vending machine at work? If you are going to consume that many calories, why not at least opt for a pastry from the bakery and a freshly brewed cup of coffee. Split the pastry with a co-worker and you can enjoy a better product and save calories at the same time. You can literally have your cake and eat it. It's all about choices and not feeling deprived while you make these choices.

Weight loss has to be a positive experience to be sustained. Thinking about *year-pounds* is your tool to success. It is your way to balance your checkbook between pleasure and weight loss, between eating and deferring. And, as you are succeeding in your weight loss, you will be eating the foods you really like, and skipping those not-so-great foods that were simply there when you were hungry. You will avoid empty calories and weight bombs that provide little enjoyment.

CHAPTER 3

SEVENTEEN KEYS TO SELF-REALIZATION AND WEIGHT LOSS, OR SEVENTEEN WAYS TO HELP YOURSELF TO A QUARTER POUND

Summary:
This chapter describes seventeen keys to unlock a successful weight loss program. Armed with a few principles and a basic understanding, you will be on your way— an expert weight loser shedding ounces and pounds—with little effort. The Contents page summarizes the key points, and it's a quick read to get the general idea. Reading each key in depth will help you understand the hows and whys. Read some. Read all. Read them in or out of order, but read them.

Key 1:   <u>*Look for small calories to give up on a regular basis.*</u>

Key 2:   <u>*Read labels, save pounds.*</u> *Seemingly, identical foods can have very different calorie content. Understand the difference between heart-healthy foods and weight control.*

Key 3:   <u>*Weigh yourself.*</u>

Key 4:   <u>*Realize hunger is your friend.*</u> *If you are full, you are not losing weight.*

Key 5:   <u>*Know yourself.*</u> *Plan to be bad. In fact, be bad to be good. Understand and work with your weaknesses. Keep snacks on hand, but select them carefully. Lighten up. Eat out once a week even though restaurants can be a poor caloric choice.*

Key 6:   *Eat more to eat less.* Skipping meals increases hunger and leads to counter-productive eating.

Key 7:   *Eat correctly.* Eat slowly. Learn "table techniques," which promote weight loss.

Key 8:   *Realize the freezer is your friend.* Made-ahead meals prevent impulse eating and save time, money, and calories. And, they are easy to prepare.

Key 9:   *Realize alcohol is not your friend, and comments on other beverages.* Despite any health claims about the benefits of a couple ounces of alcohol, the truth is, alcohol (100 calories per 1.5 ounces) stimulates the appetite, and is usually consumed with high calorie snack items. And who drinks only a couple ounces? Coffee and tea are low in calories, but what you do with them may not be. A caramel cappuccino is three hundred and fifty calories (thirty-five year-pounds).

Key 10: *Beware of deadly salads.* Croutons, nuts, seeds, and dressings change vegetables into high calorie items.

Key 11: *Beware of the vegetarian myth and the low fat fallacy.* Just because you are a vegetarian does not mean you won't be overweight. Calories are calories, whether they are from animal or plant sources. Low fat does not necessarily mean low calorie.

Key 12: *Beware of fad diets.* They just don't work over time.

Key 13: *Beware of restaurants and takeout.* No one can lose weight eating in restaurants, even eating carefully. There are all sorts of hidden calories. Nevertheless, eat out once a week, and plan to be bad.

Key 14: *Be a food snob.* Eat only foods that taste good and are worth eating, foods that are "to die for." This will increase enjoyment and decrease weight.

Key 15: *Enlist others in your quest.*

Key 16: *Exercise is a must, but easier than you think.* Losing weight actually slows metabolism and calorie burn rate. Exercise increases and promotes continuing weight loss. The calories burned by exercise add to the calories not eaten. Eating one hundred and twenty calories less a day, plus burning a hundred and twenty calories exercising, results in losing twenty-four pounds in twelve months—doubling your initial goal. Exercise can be easy, just like cutting calories. I'll show you how.

Key 17: <u>Break the rules</u>. Try different things and see what works for you. No one knows you as well as you do. When it comes to weight loss, no one is an expert or has all the answers. Everyone is different. So, within the general principles, experiment. Add your own ideas. (Maybe dessert before dinner really works for you.) A scale will be your guide to your success. Write a competing book if you want. I welcome it if it helps people lose weight.

Key 1: Look for small calories to give up on a regular basis.

In Chapter 2, I discussed the general approach to shaving calories off food while not having to give up the food entirely. The simplest approach to this is to eat less of what you are already eating or omit part of it. Leave a bite or two of your sandwich. Serve yourself a smaller portion of potatoes. Get a scoop of ice cream in a cup instead of in a cone. (A cone is really just a substitute for a cup anyway. A cup has no calories, and even the plainest cone is forty-five calories, that's four and a half pounds a year on a daily basis.) And, skip the cherry on the ice cream sundae.

Another powerful tool is to substitute one food item for another, eating the less caloric one that still tastes great and makes you happy. To do this, you need some basic knowledge about the number of calories in some of your favorite foods. Believe me, this is easy, will take only a minimal amount of time and effort, and prove to be a very powerful tool. Remember, every hundred calories saved is ten pounds a year.

A snack of raisins (two-thirds cup) is three hundred calories; grapes are only fifty-eight. *Eating grapes instead of raisins results in a savings of 242 calories. That translates into 24.2 pounds saved on a yearly basis (24.2 year-pounds).* A chicken breast is 142 calories a serving; a turkey breast is just 30, that's 11.2 *year-pounds* less. And on and on it goes—calories adding up to ounces, ounces adding up to pounds. You simply need to look around for calories to save by knowing some basic food facts.

In Appendix I, I have compiled an abbreviated list of the calorie content of a few common foods. Since each of us eats different things, you should look at numbers that apply specifically to you. The Internet has all sorts of tables and lists of the calories in common food groups including fast foods and prepared foods. Go to Google and type in "calorie content of foods," or go to the United

States Department of Agriculture Web site (*www.usda.gov*) for a list of the nutritional content of foods.

I would also suggest you consider getting a book of food contents that are readily available and inexpensive. The books have values for every food item you could imagine. And it's actually fun to look at the numbers; they will amaze you when you examine the caloric content and difference among foods. Some differences are so staggering it's almost unbelievable. Spend a few minutes looking at some of these lists. There is no need to memorize them. Just get a general idea of the differences. You can always refer to the lists as needed, and in time, caloric food contents will become second nature. By learning about caloric contents, you will find it easier to shave off those extra calories. Start to play the game "How Low Can I Go?" How many calories can you give up and still enjoy the food? This game works for both preparing and eating foods. This chart illustrates how you can save calories with a few facts and substitutions.

Weight Saving Food Choices

BETTER FOOD CHOICE *	CALORIES/ COMPARABLE SERVING SIZE	YEARLY WEIGHT SAVED BY EATING THE LOWER CALORIE ITEM ON A DAILY BASIS (*Year-pounds*)
Peanuts*	565	**5 pounds saved**
Almonds	615	
Orange*	65	**4.6 pounds saved**
Orange juice	111	
Grapefruit*	37	**5.9 pounds saved**
Grapefruit juice	96	
Peach, fresh*	37	**27.4 pounds saved**
Peaches, dried	311	

BETTER FOOD CHOICE *	CALORIES/ COMPARABLE SERVING SIZE	YEARLY WEIGHT SAVED BY EATING THE LOWER CALORIE ITEM ON A DAILY BASIS (*Year-pounds*)
Apricots, fresh*	51	3.2 pounds saved
Apricots, dried	83	
Grapes*	58	24.2 pounds saved
Raisins	300	
Banana*	105	3 pounds saved
Papaya*	117	1.8 pounds saved
Mango	135	
Turkey breast*	30	11.2 pounds saved
Chicken breast	142	
Pork loin*	166	9.1 pounds saved
Beef loin	257	
	NOTE Below: Ribs are the reverse, though both are high calorie.	
Pork ribs	397	
Beef ribs*	362	3.5 pounds saved

Lose the dried fruit. Lose the beef. And lose the weight. Have your cake and eat it, but maybe without the icing! Or, maybe just half a slice.

Perhaps you want some nuts because they are now in vogue as one of the "good foods." Would you settle for peanuts (Calories: 565 per 3.5 ounces) instead of almonds (Calories: 615 per 3.5 ounces)? You will save fifty calories, or *five year-pounds*. **It's all about choices.**

Remember, that while it's good to make choices that save calories, it's best to do it happily and be satisfied, or you will not persist with your diet. If almonds make you happy and peanuts don't, go with the almonds and have less of something else or fewer almonds.

Another example. Orange juice is much more caloric than an orange. Why? Because it takes two to three oranges to make a glass of juice. So, settle for an orange instead of orange juice and you save calories. Intuitive, but generally not thought about.

A quick look at the previous chart may point out some interesting thoughts about other choices that may also surprise you. Look at the difference between dried and fresh fruit. Once you understand the concept of looking for calorie savings, while still enjoying what you are eating, you will find other ways to shave off calories and cheat the scale. (Check out the appendixes for examples and more ideas.)

Just like selecting foods to save calories, you can shave calories and lose weight by careful preparation of the foods you choose. Fat is nine calories per gram of weight; carbohydrates and protein are four, less than half. We will deal with the high protein/low carb diets later, but for now, if you cut down the fat in a recipe you will shave off calories and pounds.

Every tablespoon of oil or fat is one hundred and twenty calories; that's twelve *year-pounds*, which are two and a half bags of flour. It does not matter if this is saturated fat like Crisco or butter, or unsaturated fat like olive oil or canola. Remember, we are talking about weight, not heart health; weight is calories, pure and simple. Olive oil is certainly far better for your cholesterol and your heart than a heavily saturated shortening, but to your waistline, calories are calories and fat is fat. So, the patient who told me she was upset because she didn't lose weight when she substituted olive oil for butter, just didn't understand.

Here is a perfect example of how to shave calories, or more to the point, weight. I recently wanted to make a meatless Spanish rice entrée with lots of vegetables. The original recipe called for a quarter cup of olive oil to sauté the vegetables. That is four hundred and eighty calories. I used two tablespoons of olive oil and added a little nonfat stock when I needed more liquid to soften the vegetables. This saved about two hundred and forty calories; forty calories per person. That's a third of the way to your one hundred and twenty calories per day, twelve pounds per year. You can apply this cooking method to a stir-fry dish as well. Use only a minimal amount of oil, add the vegetables in their natural state and their juices will provide the liquid necessary to sauté the meat or chicken. Almost all stir-fry recipes call for more oil than is needed. In fact, you may find this is true with a majority of recipes.

Remember, each tablespoon of oil not used saves you a hundred and twenty calories (your goal for the day). Your job is to seek out and do away with fats and oils. If you are baking, ripe bananas or applesauce can be substituted for oil in many recipes. Yes, there are healthy fats such as fish oil and fats found in certain nuts, but remember your waistline is a calorie meter, not a health gauge. All oil contains the same calories. When your weight goes down, your health level goes up, even if you are a bit short on fish oil and almond butter.

 Key 2: Read labels, save pounds.

Muffin A

Nutrition Facts	
Serving Size 2 oz (57g)	
Servings Per Container 6	

Calories 200	
Calories from Fat 100	

Amount Per Serving	% Daily Value
Total Fat 11g	17%
Saturated Fat 2g	10%
Trans Fat 0g	
Cholesterol 40 mg	14%
Sodium 220 mg	9%
Total Carbohydrate 24g	8%
Dietary Fiber 0g	0%
Sugars 13g	
Protein 3g	

Vitamin A 2%	Vitamin C 0%
Thiamine 6%	Riboflavin 8%
Niacin 6%	Calcium 2%
Iron 6%	Folic Acid 2%

Muffin B

Nutrition Facts	
Serving Size 71g (2.5 oz or 1 muffin)	
Servings Per Container 3	

Amount Per Serving	
Calories 180	
Calories from Fat 25	

	% Daily Value
Total Fat 3g	5%
Saturated Fat 1g	5%
Trans Fat 0%	
Cholesterol 20 mg	7%
Sodium 350 mg	15%
Total Carbohydrate 38g	13%
Dietary Fiber 3g	12%
Sugars 20g	
Protein 3g	

Vitamin A 2%	Vitamin C 0%
Thiamine 2%	Riboflavin 2%
Niacin 6%	Calcium 2%
Iron 2%	Folic Acid 0%

On the previous page are two examples of information contained on the nutrition facts food labels that you probably do not read or are reading incorrectly.
These labels are on packaged food items to help you understand what's inside
… supposedly. These labels contain all sorts of information, too much, in
fact. Serving size. Calories. Fat content. Amount of saturated fat and trans fat.
Percentages of daily requirements of things like iron and calcium, and so on.
There is so much information that most people ignore the label. You don't have
time to check it all out on every product or you will never get your shopping
done. *There are two simple facts on every label that are key to helping you lose
weight—serving size and calories.*

Remember, we are talking about weight loss and calories, not cardiac health
(fats and cholesterol) or insulin secretion (sugars and carbohydrates). These will
improve indirectly as you lose weight. So, initially, don't labor over the carbohydrate and fat contents. You can learn to analyze and use these parameters
later as you get more sophisticated in your approach to nutrition. *First things
first—serving size and calories. And even these can be tricky.*

*Serving size seems like an easy place to begin. However, this is a treacherous
and slippery slope.* You need to be very careful not to be deceived.

Note the two muffin labels. Both packages contain three muffins. Brand
A muffins are much larger than Brand B muffins. They are quite tempting in
that when you look at the calories per serving size, they seem to be only twenty
calories more than Brand B (200 versus 180) as listed on the label. The *serving
size* of each product as listed is about the same (2 oz. for Brand A, 2.5oz. for
Brand B). So again, you would assume there is only a twenty-calorie difference
between the Brand B muffin and its super-sized big brother, Brand A.

However, note that the *number of servings per container is different (disguised
by where "Amount Per Serving" is placed on muffin A's label).* Brand A contains
three muffins, but six servings. Brand B contains three muffins and three servings. Brand B muffins are each one serving. Each Brand A muffin, however, is
considered *two* servings. So the *calories per serving* of the Brand A muffin actually
represent the calories in *half* a muffin, and who eats half a muffin? This means
that each Brand A muffin is really four hundred calories (*forty year-pounds*),
not two hundred as you would first think. Brand A muffin looks bigger and *is*
bigger, and you will be too if you eat it. Whether or not to eat the bigger Brand
A muffin is up to you. If it is "to die for," eat it and enjoy it, but do so know-

ingly and realize the consequences. Consider eating half of Brand A muffin, or a Brand B muffin instead. Better yet, eat a piece of fruit.

This type of *confusing labeling is everywhere*, not just on muffin packaging. When we buy a product such as a beverage or a bag of chips, we assume the calories listed on the label are for the unit. This is not always the case. A bottle of a popular iced tea lists one hundred calories per serving. However, the bottle contains two servings. So that's two hundred calories per bottle, or twenty *year-pounds*. Few of us drink half a can or bottle with our lunch, so realize you are consuming two hundred calories, not one hundred.

So much for starting with the seemingly simple concept of serving size. We have already peeked at the calorie area of the label above, but let's look at it in more detail. Again, I urge you to look at calories in terms of *year-pounds*, the measure of what you would gain eating an item every day for a year, over and above what you normally eat. As opposed to trying to picture a calorie, this gives you a concrete idea about how good or bad a food is in terms of your weight. Again, obtain this value by simply dividing the calories per serving by ten. So, let's proceed and see how simple choices can save you ounces and pounds.

Many seemingly similar foods are quite different in calorie content. Here are just a couple examples. We'll start with a slice of whole wheat bread. Simple enough. Two loaves on the shelf look very much alike. However, National Brand A is ninety calories a slice, while Brand B is only seventy. This is a savings of twenty calories per slice. Since most of us eat two slices that's a forty-calorie difference, which is four *year-pounds*, almost a bag of flour. Of note is the fact that a slice of Brand A weighs thirty-eight grams, while Brand B is only thirty-one grams a slice. This accounts for much of the calorie difference, so there is really nothing magical about Brand B. Since, however, we eat our bread in slices, not grams, the calories saved by eating Brand B are real.

Now, let's compare two chocolate sandwich cookies. Cookies made by Company X are 200 calories for three cookies (37gm). Company Y's cookies are only 160 calories for three cookies (34gm). Again, some of the difference is in the weight of the cookies, but we eat cookies by number, not grams. So go for Company Y's cookies and save four *year-pounds*, almost another bag of flour.

How about frozen entrées designed to help with weight loss? As an example, let's look at Salisbury steak with potatoes and vegetables: Company Q, 200 calories. Company R, 270 calories. Company S, 350 calories. Which would you choose? Now in all fairness, Company Q's meal is only nine ounces and the other two are twelve and a half ounces. But you eat by container not ounces, and even if you eliminate Company Q, there still is a significant difference between Company R and Company S—eight *year-pounds* in fact. By looking carefully, you can find a prepared entrée with fewer calories. If, however, the less caloric version is not to your liking, eat the higher calorie one and find your one hundred and twenty calories a day elsewhere.

So, by simply choosing between brands of three items (your bread, your cookie, and your frozen entrée), you have already saved sixteen year-pounds, which is twenty-five percent more than your quarter pound a week goal.

 ### Key 3: Weigh yourself.

As discussed earlier, there is no absolute calorie per day goal set by my method. This is simply too difficult a number to arrive at for any given individual—that is what being *individual* means. So, how do you know if you're winning or losing by making choices like those above? The obvious answer is to weigh yourself. But there are important things to consider about this simple process.

There is a truism. If you never gain back the weight you lose, you will eventually reach your weight loss goal even if you lose only miniscule amounts of weight at a time. The key is to move forward, not backward, no matter how slowly. Eventually, you will weigh what you want. This is where the scale comes in. It is very hard to judge weight, and emotionally difficult to admit to any weight gain.

"I didn't gain weight, my pants shrank. I'm not too heavy, I'm just too short for my weight." The scale acts as your impartial partner giving you a factual reference point. The very factual nature of the scale is the reason why some overweight people avoid using it.

"The scale is just so uncaring. It doesn't care that I am stressed and eating chocolate because of it." I can't tell you how many of my overweight patients simply do not own or want to own a scale. *In truth, a scale gives facts, not judgments. Only you are judgmental.*

The scale doesn't say, "You shouldn't have had that piece of pie every day this week." You do. The scale only indicates you now weigh two pounds more. This is a fact, not a criticism. Therefore, if you use the data it provides constructively, the scale is a valuable aid and will become your friend, not your foe. The uncaring nature of the scale should be viewed as a plus.

The key to making the scale your friend is realizing it provides numbers, not criticism. If your weight is up, it is nice to know so you can correct the course before you have gained a huge amount of weight.

How do I weigh myself and how often?

There are some tips to using your weight advisor (a.k.a. "your scale") correctly. Weigh yourself in the morning before you have eaten. Weigh yourself with your clothes off, or in the same clothes to avoid variation in clothing weight. A digital scale or balance beam scale (like the one your doctor uses) is a good idea. They are more accurate than typical bathroom scales, but this is not critical.

I suggest weighing yourself only once a week, unless you've done some unusual eating and you need a reality check as to where you are. Weighing yourself too often is oppressive and can be upsetting; it can also give you the wrong impression.

Though not perfect, the scale gives you a benchmark of how well you are doing or how much more you need to do. It provides a definite number, but not an interpretation of what is going on at any one moment. Weight can vary considerably and rapidly for reasons other than calories. So any one reading that is higher can upset you because you have reduced calories, yet your weight is up. If you are consistently reducing calories, the number on the scale will almost certainly go down the next reading. The scale is very helpful by the nature of its exactness, but only helpful, not the end all.

Despite the gravitational accuracy of a scale, any weight is not an exact measure of what is going on in any one person at any one time. Be happy if your weight is less than it was a week ago, but don't panic if it's higher. Scales are best at providing trends.

Many things can affect weight. Water retention and level of hydration can temporarily increase weight. A high intake of salt results in water retention that can rapidly increase weight several pounds in a day. This weight gain resolves when one goes back on a low salt intake.

For women, water retention often occurs with the menstrual cycle. Again, this can give a false impression of what is going on. For this reason, I suggest not weighing just before menstruation. Having eaten all day, or not having gone to the bathroom can also affect weight.

Remember we are looking for long-term results, not day-to-day variations. That's why I suggested weighing yourself only once a week. Weighing yourself more often may cause you to focus on short-term rather than long-term goals and this will probably drive you crazy. However, I suggest weighing yourself more often if you are concerned that due to repeated indiscretions you have gained weight. This will confirm if it is true and allow you to correct your course sooner while you are still at a manageable weight gain. Remember, each day of extra calories calls for action, and the sooner you correct the problem, the better. For some reason it always seems easier to gain rather than lose weight. Life is just not fair.

In addition to weighing yourself regularly but not excessively, I suggest setting a "red line weight" so you can avoid the "Panic Zone." The red line represents your maximum weight, a line you will never cross or never go beyond. This reference point is adjusted downward in comfortable increments as you lose weight. *Just like everything else, set modest attainable goals and meet them, rather than shoot for the moon and fall short.* There will be times when you will go off your weight loss plan and probably gain some weight. No guilt, just a fact. If you are still below your red line weight, small changes in consumption will get you back on track. In fact, you do not need to change from your regular plan as you are below the red line and will be losing weight again as you resume your plan to lose your four ounces a week. You will simply take a little longer to reach your goal.

If you are above the red line, I recommend you be more aggressive and do what it takes to get below the line as quickly as you are able. You can then resume your regular, more gradual plan. Why do I say this since with your regular plan you will eventually drop below the red line anyway? Being above the line poses a psychological problem. With each indiscretion it gets easier and easier to allow yourself to cross the line and stay above it, and harder to get back below it. Initially, getting back in control will involve only a few pounds. Left to multiply, the pounds increase and the physical and psychological difficulty associated with losing the weight increases. Seeking to lose three to five pounds is manageable. Ten pounds is formidable. Twenty is a task. You are now in the "Panic Zone," fearing defeat. You can still do it an ounce at a time, but with each increase, it will take longer. This may seem daunting. It is better not to go there than have to come back. Staying below the line also means you do not have to focus on your weight all the time. You have a "cushion" of a few pounds before you have to work harder to lose weight rather than simply stay on your regular program. You do not have to be preoccupied every minute of the day with your weight. You can correct small, occasional indiscretions subliminally. You are now free from the shackles of perpetually dieting. You are thinking and behaving like a thin person.

I feel it is very important to make the scale your friend, not your enemy. Its very simplicity makes it a valuable and sophisticated tool. It automatically factors in food intake, exercise, and metabolic rate. The scale is your guide to a successful journey through the jungle of calories. It helps you avoid having to keep track of and list every bit of food and drink. It is your calorie meter telling you if you are on the path to success.

 ## Key 4: Realize hunger is your friend.

In addition to the scale, you have a built-in weight monitor—your stomach. *You cannot lose weight and feel completely full. Despite the claims of some diets, you cannot eat all the calories you want, feel full, and lose weight. Ideally, if you are losing weight, you should always feel a little less than full, even after you have finished a meal. This does not need to be unpleasant.* I said a little less than full, not ravenous, or deprived. Once again it comes down to attitude and understanding. *Make hunger your friend, not your enemy.* If you are feeling hungry, you can be satisfied you are losing weight and meeting your goal. After a while, feeling full will actually feel uncomfortable. Thin people automatically tune into this. Being a little empty also means that if a particularly good snack presents itself, you can enjoy it and not go off the track as much as if you were already full. No guilt, and minimal work to recover.

Another aspect of hunger is using it to decide when to eat. *Thin people eat when they are hungry. Heavy people eat by the clock.*

Many years ago, when I was in college taking a psychology class, I was struck by a fascinating study. A group of heavy and thin students gathered in a classroom containing a refrigerator filled with food. The students were given a long test and told they could eat whatever and whenever they wanted. Unbeknownst to those assembled, the clock in the classroom, altered to run fast, showed noon when it was only 11:00 AM. Interestingly, at what seemed like noon by the clock (noon being the traditional lunch hour), the overweight students went to the refrigerator to get something to eat. The thin ones waited until the clock showed 1:00 or 1:30 to eat. They were eating because of hunger, not because the clock indicated noon. So, hunger has two benefits. It tells you when to eat and when to stop ... *if you listen.*

While being hungry is good, there are some tricks to help you feel comfortable even when you are hungry. You can fool your stomach into thinking it is fuller than it is. Drink a lot of water, especially when you are hungry or eating. Water fills up the stomach and has no calories. Eating a lot of fiber and roughage also fills up the stomach, especially in combination with water. Salads are great for this as long as you watch those high calorie dressings, croutons, nut toppings, etc. "Bulking up" is in fact how some diet drinks work. They are loaded with fiber that has few calories, and makes the dieter feel full. Eating slowly also gives your stomach time to register what it has consumed and signals the brain to halt intake. Drinking water between bites of food fills you up *and* slows you down at the same time.

So, be hungry and be happy—happy you are losing weight.

 Key 5: Know yourself.

As I have said, set reasonable goals and meet them. Avoid the frustration of failure by not setting overly optimistic goals and falling short. When looking to shave off calories, do not give up so many of your favorite foods that you become unhappy. Start by eating less of what you normally would and enjoy. Half a dessert, a small piece of cheese, a half glass of wine. Try splitting an entrée with your significant other or a friend. In time, you will be willing to give up some foods entirely, if you do it on your own terms. Eventually you may be able to give up those tempting desserts and settle for a bite of someone else's treat. You may be happy with just a taste of wine. Perhaps you can bring yourself to do the same with appetizers and snacks.

However, there is a possible pitfall to tastes and sips. Sometimes it is easier not to eat something than to try being temperate once you have tasted it. Food stimulates the appetite for more food. Do you have the willpower to eat a limited amount? Or do you find eating nothing at all is easier? Can you eat just one potato chip? Only you can decide. Maybe you need to eat a *small* bag of potato chips and give up something else, or maybe you would be happier with light potato chips made with Olestra, a soy fat substitute with many fewer calories ' than most other cooking oils.

Even if you cannot eat only a nibble or a bite to satisfy your tastebuds, there is still hope. Once again, I offer you the nickel and dime approach to accumulating dollars. The quarter-pound weight loss plan.

Start with your usual portion of a particular food. Next time, decrease the amount. Divide it where you feel comfortable, eat the reduced portion, and leave the rest. (Contrary to what your parents told you, there are few rewards for being a member of the "clean plate club.") Continue to shave off portion sizes and calories until you reach a point that is comfortable, but not further reducible. Over time you will serve up a comfortably reduced portion of food, and shave calories even if you cannot give up the food item entirely. Remember, as long as you are eating less than before, you are losing weight.

Plan to be bad. In fact, you need to be bad to be good. Part of knowing yourself is planning to be bad, which actually allows you to be good. What do I mean by this? We all get cravings. As mentioned before, you need to think of hunger as your friend. If you are hungry, you are losing weight. In the right mental state, you can actually enjoy feeling a little hungry rather than feeling overly full. But it is normal at times when you are hungry to have cravings and desires to nibble and snack.

Rather than assume you will always rise above cravings, I suggest you admit that you will almost certainly have eating urges that you will answer, even if you are actively engaged in a weight loss program. Rather than deny these urges, why not plan to be bad? Desperately scavenging through cupboards looking for a snack can be a very high calorie event unless you have prepared. So, I insist you go to the store and spend lots of time picking out some tasty snacks to keep in your cupboard. The key, however, is to be "bad" not "stupid."

Select snacks that are appealing, but as low as possible in calorie content. You want cookies? Go for it. But check the label and choose accordingly. Try for one that is satisfying, but relatively low in calories. Chocolate? Go for the dark if you are willing. Dark chocolate contains less fat and fewer calories. Popcorn? Get the reduced fat and calorie type. But do remember, *low fat does not always mean fewer calories. Check the label.*

Low fat is a good idea for general health. But remember, regardless of the source, it's still the total calories that count toward weight loss. So watch not only what you eat, but how much. *You can gain lots of weight by eating too much low fat food. Also, remember you have choices to make even with good foods without fat.*

In the table on page **20** (*Weight Saving Food Choices*), note that dried fruit, which seems healthy and contains little fat, still has calories. Moreover, there are choices among various dried fruits. Raisins are three hundred calories per two-thirds cup. A better choice is dried apricots at eighty-three calories per ten halves. Or, instead of raisins, try fresh grapes weighing in at fifty-eight calories. *Eating grapes on a daily basis instead of raisins saves about twenty-four pounds of weight a year.*

So, do try to be good and not snack excessively. But when you do answer the call, be stocked with better food items than you might have found if you had not prepared and made intelligent choices in advance. Instead of those stale cookies left in the back of the pantry, enjoy the fresh low calorie ones you bought. Being prepared is the key. (This same principle applies not only to snacks, but also to unplanned meals discussed in Key 8.)

Another part of being bad is eating out occasionally. Yes, I have a whole section about fattening and high calorie restaurant food. It is almost impossible to eat at restaurants and not overshoot your daily calories. So, why do I suggest dining out, perhaps once a week or every other week?

As I previously mentioned, eating is more than a means of staying alive. It is a social event. It is a reward. It can be an art form and a hobby. It is a pleasant experience. Just as you cannot give up all your favorite foods and remain happy and on course, you must not give up all the fun of dining out.

During the week, you work diligently to simplify your foods, reduce portions, and lose weight. Come Saturday go out and relax, and enjoy the fun of eating some treats in a restaurant. This will prevent you from feeling deprived and make it possible to stay on your program without being angry that you are always giving things up. Go out and have fun, but don't be foolish. Try to pick foods you will enjoy, but are lower in calories. Would a baked potato do instead of fries? If the fries are "to die for," enjoy them and find calories elsewhere to shave, either at this meal or another. Are you willing to share an appetizer, an entrée, a dessert? Do you need dessert? Are the desserts at this restaurant really that good? Maybe sorbet instead of ice cream. Enjoy yourself, that's why you're out, but eat knowingly and choose food carefully. (More about this under Key 13.)

Key 6: Eat more to eat less.

We have already talked a little about urges and cravings. When trying to lose weight, it is helpful not to respond to urges for treats, snacks, fattening foods, etc. *Some people try to skip meals entirely in an attempt to cut down calories and improve weight loss. Unfortunately, this often results in just the opposite effect.*

Your goal is to eat less, lose weight, and enjoy the feeling of being modestly hungry, realizing this is your signal you are losing weight. The key word is *modestly* hungry. Excessive hunger leads to foolish acts of frustration. If you eat a moderate breakfast and then nothing until dinnertime, chances are you will arrive home ravenous. As you enter the kitchen, hunger urges increase. You simply cannot wait until dinner is on the table. Nibbles will be calling to you. A handful of crackers, a piece of bread, a cookie, a piece of cheese. Perhaps with a beer or a glass of wine. One beer and four crackers and a slice of cheese are about three hundred and fifty calories; thirty-five *year-pounds*. This will take one and a quarter hours of moderate walking to burn off. These are wasted calories that are not even fully enjoyed, just eaten quickly to stave off hunger pangs until dinner is on the table.

A much better approach is to eat a modest lunch and perhaps a small mid afternoon snack of something satisfying, but not too caloric. (Suggestion: a nonfat yogurt and some fruit, a few peanuts or almonds, a piece of fruit, a small piece of low fat cheese, etc.) When you get home, your eating will be more controlled. Remember, it is total calories that count, not how you divide them. Overeating negates the skipping of a meal. Conversely, grazing—eating frequent small portions of food throughout the day—does not need to lead to weight gain as long as the total calories eaten are within your daily goal. This method of eating also avoids large insulin surges, thus helping to promote weight loss and general health.

Eat enough at dinner to help curb evening snacking desires. Dinner is a meal where people often try to limit their intake in an attempt to lose weight. "I'll just have a yogurt or a salad." This often stems from indiscretion at lunch. This is a fine idea if you can limit dinner calories and still feel satisfied. But remember, if you leave the table too hungry, and as a result snack all night, you may defeat the purpose of eating fewer calories at dinner.

Key 7: Eat correctly.

Since we were just discussing dinner issues, I will use this opportunity to talk about some eating principles that are simple and intuitive, but often not followed. These principles apply to all meals, but I chose dinner because in the United States it is generally the largest meal.

Here are some helpful eating techniques.

First, *choose plates and glasses on the small side*. This helps enforce portion size. We tend to eat guided by the apparent size of a portion. *A soft-boiled egg in a china eggcup looks like an elegant light breakfast. One scrambled egg on a full-sized plate gets lost and calls for a side of bacon and some flapjacks!* Years ago, there was a hamburger chain that shaped the burgers like a donut with a hole in the center. This caused the burger to stick out of the bun, giving the impression it was larger than it was, a seeming bargain compared to those tiny burgers sold elsewhere. In truth, no more beef, just perception.

Next, *eat slowly*. It takes time for the brain to receive a signal from the stomach that you have eaten and are full. There is inertia at work here. If you eat faster than signals get to the brain, there is a good chance you will eat more than you really need to be comfortably full. (Or should I say still feel pleasantly hungry?) Chew your food slowly; take your time. If you insist on chewing and eating quickly, or must because of your lifestyle, stop eating after you have consumed a predetermined portion of food. Stop after consuming the portion even if you still feel hungry. Wait five minutes. Agree you will eat more only if you are still hungry. You will be amazed how many times you will find yourself full at that point, and eat no more, or at least eat less at a later time.

Drink plenty of water, still or bubbly. Have a glass before dinner. This helps fill you up. Have another with your meal. Sips between bites will slow your eating and help you feel full. Adequate water intake is very good for you.

Do not put serving dishes on the table. Put food portions on a plate and bring the plate to the table. Not having serving dishes or a breadbasket on the table prevents idle eating and nibbling. Somehow, when we sit at the table talking and relaxing, our hands guide themselves to the serving platter or the breadbasket and help themselves to more food. So much for portion control. If you want more food and feel it's within your calorie allotment, get up and help yourself. This should be a conscious decision, not the inadvertent action of idle hands. Getting up from the table has several beneficial aspects. It gives you some time to reconsider if you really need more. Is more food really "to die for?" It also gives your brain time to get its message from the stomach, helping you make this decision. Lastly, walking to get a second helping affords a small amount of exercise and burns some calories!

Two exceptions to food on the table are a pitcher of water and a bowl of salad, assuming the salad is made correctly, which will be discussed later in the book. Other than this, hike for the second helping.

 ## Key 8: Realize the freezer is your friend.

Now that we have discussed how you are going to eat, *I would like to address what you are eating, how you prepare it, and how not to have to prepare it.*

For many people, dealing with dinner is a big issue. Usually the largest meal of the day, dinner is the most damaging when it comes to consuming unneeded calories. Many people are busy and feel they just do not have time to make a nutritious, calorie-controlled, tasty dinner at home. Actually, it is easier than you think. *Just as you need to eat more to eat less (Key 6), you need to cook more to cook less.*

For many of us, dinner preparation needs to be fast. Our lives are just so busy. Lured by takeout Chinese, pizza, and supermarket prepared foods, we hope to free up time in our overcommitted lives. Many of these are high calorie items, even the ones that seem innocent.

Chinese food, for example, is cooked with significant amounts of oil. Fried rice is 363 calories per cup, and a serving of lemon chicken is 412, or 41.2 *year-pounds*. Italian entrées are caloric as well. A plain cheese pizza ranges from 210 to 290 calories *per slice*. And, how many of us eat just one slice? Vegetarian pizza and pepperoni pizza range from 220 to 310 calories per slice. So, if you down three slices, you're dealing with 87 *year-pounds*. What about that rotisserie chicken you brought home from the supermarket? Seems healthy enough. But a rotisserie chicken can run as high as 500 calories per serving. If you are careful and eat just a quarter of a chicken—white meat only, no wing, and no skin—you can get away with about 170 calories. Not bad. However, if you throw in a side of baked beans and potato salad, you add about 630 calories, or 63 *year-pounds*. So, if you stay with just the chicken and a simple salad, you at least have a chance.

So, how does one deal with time constraints and the need to eat dinner? Takeout or dining out in a restaurant is viewed as the solution. But is it? *I will show you how it's quicker making dinner at home than waiting in line at the supermarket or eating in a restaurant. (Remember to include getting there and back.) More importantly, it will almost certainly be less caloric.* Eating at home will also probably be less expensive so you can save some money to put toward your weekly evening out. Save the calories and your money. Is the fast food, which is not always so fast, "to die for?" Why not hold out for food that is *really* to die for. Make dining out a special event, not just a quick fix, which is neither quick nor a fix for your weight.

So, what is the solution? Flash Fish and Quick Chick.

Preparing low calorie meals at home is not that difficult or time-consuming. It simply requires some planning. *You need to make more to make less.* What do I mean by this? I suggest buying food in bulk and setting aside portions for future use. This is why I make the comment that the freezer is your friend. I commonly hear people say they do not shop at warehouse stores because they live alone or with one other person. They feel the quantities sold at these stores are too large for their needs. That's the point. *The idea is to cook in quantity and carefully set aside the extra food for future meals.* Such stored food makes quick, low calorie, tasty meals, and saves money as well.

Let me give you an example. My wife and I have busy schedules. We like to eat carefully and efficiently. We find eating out time consuming and expensive, and the food is often not healthy. The same goes for takeout.

Therefore, we evolved a system as follows. Let's say we are grilling salmon. Instead of cooking only a small portion, we will usually grill two large fillets weighing about four and a half pounds total. After grilling the fish, we set aside what we plan to eat during the next day or two. Then we cut the rest into individual portions and wrap it carefully in plastic wrap. We place these portions in a freezer bag, date, and freeze for future use. Carefully handled fish can be kept in the freezer two to three months. (Low oil fish up to six months.) Frozen fish that is thawed and then cooked loses its texture. Cooked first, fish keeps beautifully. When you are ready for a fish dinner, remove a packaged portion from the freezer and thaw by placing it in the refrigerator that morning, or immerse the plastic bag in a bowl of lukewarm water until thawed. Microwave thawing tends to cook the fish and ruin the texture.

What do we do with the fish when thawed? We eat it at room temperature, perhaps on a salad. It makes a great "tuna" salad (with low fat mayonnaise). Spicy fish cakes, lightly sautéed rather than fried, are one of my favorites. *So, by cooking just once in volume and using the freezer wisely, we have prepared many main courses that need only a quick salad (fresh or pre-packaged) or a vegetable to complete the meal. Dinner in less than ten minutes.*

Chicken breasts bought in bulk are an alternative to salmon. Grill the chicken breasts right alongside fish when preparing future meals. Store in individually wrapped packages, date, and place in freezer for an easy meal later. The more food you precook, and carefully package and store, the more no-effort low calorie meals you have available.

Another of my favorite meals is poached rather than grilled chicken. Poaching chicken provides a base for an almost infinite number of dishes. Chicken prepared this way and then frozen remains extremely moist and tender. While it is very tasty, the taste is not overpowering, so poached chicken is great in almost any dish with just about any sauce.

Here's how it's done. Start with ten to twelve skinless, boneless chicken breasts. Rinse the chicken breasts and place into a large stockpot. Add cold water to cover the chicken by one and a half inches. Heat to a boil, and then reduce to a simmer. (When boiling meat or poultry, albuminous particles of protein are released, forming a scum on the surface. Do not stir the contents of the stockpot, the clouding particles will become part of the broth and mar its appearance.) Skim off the rising froth until the broth is almost clear, and then add cut up vegetables and spices as you like. If vegetables are included at the beginning, they will interfere with skimming. The vegetables can be those that are past their prime for salads. We like celery with tops and carrots, no potatoes. To this, we add sliced onion, parsley, a bay leaf, and spices. We like garlic powder, lemon pepper, and regular pepper.

Cover the pot and turn the heat to low so the chicken barely simmers for one hour. Then turn the heat off and let the pot stand covered for another hour. At this point, there are many options.

Remove a portion of the broth, vegetables, and chicken to eat that day and the next as chicken soup. Take the remaining chicken and package it into small freezer bags, usually two or three breasts to a bag. Put these small packages into a larger freezer bag, date it, and freeze. The remaining broth can be strained of vegetables and frozen in small containers to use in sauces in the future. To prepare a meal, thaw the chicken. Serve on a salad, or as a stir-fry, or make into tacos, or use in just about any recipe that calls for cooked chicken. You have just prepared five to six meals for two people with almost no effort, and you used your tired, old vegetables in the process.

You can accomplish this simple task of poaching chicken while eating Sunday breakfast and enjoying the paper. In fact, you have made several meals without really setting aside any specific time to cook. By preparing foods this way several times a month, you are ahead of immediate consumption, and even have plenty for entertaining. You have also saved money in the process by buying in bulk, and putting together meals in a few minutes negates the need for takeout in an attempt to save time.

As I said earlier, you need to make more to make less. The corollary is that the freezer is your friend. No more last minute takeout or pizzas. No more stopping by the grocery store on the way home for a main entrée. It's all in your freezer. Keep plenty of salad greens and fresh vegetables in the refrigerator, and a lovely dinner can be ready in ten minutes.

Here is another tip regarding quick and easy food preparation. As an alternative to already prepared fast foods that are generally higher in fat and salt—and not always fast, particularly if you get stuck in rush hour on the way to the restaurant or market—consider purchasing a contact grill that cooks rapidly on both sides. An example is the George Forman grill. This is an inexpensive item and cooks fish, chicken and frozen turkey burgers in minutes. Cleanup is fast and easy. When you come home from work and have almost no time for dinner, put something on the grill. While it's cooking, plop a few handfuls of pre-washed salad greens on a plate and dinner is ready in about fifteen minutes. That's less time than it takes to wait in line for takeout or eat at a restaurant. It's also considerably healthier and cheaper.

While we're on the subject of food preparation and the freezer, I would like to make a few more suggestions. Lunch is often a meal when people get sloppy or lose focus. A quick takeout or a pre-made sandwich loaded with cheese, mayonnaise, etcetera is often a less than fantastic eating experience, and usually filled with lots of calories. Instead, bring a salad or leftovers from a previous meal. I know this takes time to prepare when you are already rushing against the clock, but I offer it as an easy alternative. Or, pick up some low calorie frozen meals, which abound in the freezer section of the supermarket. They are good alternatives to takeout Chinese, Mexican, or pizza. Chosen carefully, frozen meals are tasty, low cal, and even reasonable in terms of salt content. Wait for a sale on your favorite brand and stock up. Put them in your freezer and use as needed. They cost less than most fast foods and are usually lower in calories. Calorie controlled frozen meals often taste as good as "food brought in," and they generally take only six to ten minutes to prepare. This is less time than you waste foraging for food-to-go. You can use the time saved to take a walk at lunch, burning a few calories along the way.

A few precautions regarding frozen meals: *While some frozen meals are a calorie bargain,* not all low calorie meals are as low as you might think, and some regular frozen dinners can be a real calorie bomb. Note chart below.*

*National Brand A Herb Roasted Chicken	180 calories (18 *year-pounds*)
National Brand B Herb Roasted Chicken	530 calories (53 *year-pounds*)
National Brand A Four Cheese Pizza	400 calories (40 *year-pounds*)
National Brand A Teriyaki Steak Bowl	340 calories (34 *year-pounds*)

So, read the labels and compare. Also, some frozen meals are high in sodium for those who need to watch their intake. Again, read the labels and compare.

Key 9: Realize alcohol is not your friend, and comments on other beverages.

Some studies indicate that alcohol in moderation may be good for you. A glass of red wine daily may lower the risk of heart disease. Many of my patients took this as a green light to pop the cork for medicinal purposes even if they were not wine drinkers in the past. *There is definitely some evidence that wine, or any alcohol, may have some beneficial effects, but will not help you lose weight.* A glass of wine, a beer, or a simple mixed drink has at least 100 to 200 calories. *Two drinks a day are at least 20 to 40 year-pounds.* A mai tai is at a minimum 260 calories *per drink.* You do the math. In addition to considerations of calories, alcohol is an appetite stimulant. How often do you nibble some snacks when you have your wine or beer? Enough said.

I am not totally opposed to your having a drink if it is important to you. In keeping with my approach, I want you to be happy with the weight loss process. I just ask that you be aware, count the calories, and be sure the drink is "to die for." If so, enjoy it and even the nibbles, and look for calories to discard elsewhere. If you can go without, you will save at minimum, ten pounds of calories per year, and probably more. If giving up alcohol is too large a commitment, perhaps you could opt for several abstinent days a week, and enjoy your wine perhaps even more on the remaining ones. In keeping with making this a pleasurable experience, note the following. If you drink a half bottle of $10 wine a day, you can afford to drink a half bottle of $20 wine every other day for the same cost. Better wine, fewer calories over time. Win-win.

One quick note while I am on the subject of beverages. Non-alcoholic drinks may not be your friends either. Your morning cup of black coffee or tea is zero calories, but with sugar (two teaspoons), it's 30 calories. A café latte with skim milk is around 160 calories, but with low fat milk, it's 220 calories, and with whole milk, 260 calories. A caramel cappuccino can run 350 calories, and a large hot chocolate with whipped cream can be almost 900 big ones! *Ninety year-pounds.* Is it "to die for?"

 Key 10: Beware of deadly salads.

There are salads and then there are salads. A basic garden salad of greens and vegetables has very few calories. Add some diet dressing or simply a splash of balsamic vinegar and you're still okay. But drench the salad in regular dressing and start adding salad bar goodies like shredded cheese, nuts, croutons, and bacon bits, and a new creature evolves: *The Deadly Salad.* This is why fast food restaurant salads may sound like a good idea, but may be higher in calories than some other entrées. *It all depends what is on and in the salad.* Note the following examples:

Dinner salad	89 calories
With 2 Tbsp. fat free ranch dressing ... add	+137
With 2 Tbsp. regular ranch dressing ... add	+237
Croutons/cup ... add	+122
Honey nut roasted nut topping/Tbsp ... add	+40
Bacon bits/Tbsp.... add	+33
Shredded cheddar cheese/Tbsp.... add	+33
(*Remember, a tablespoon is not much cheese*)	
National chain taco salad*	610
National chain mixed salad*	690
National chain mandarin style chicken salad*	730

*A fully loaded national chain cheeseburger seems like a bargain at 560 calories

A relative of a deadly salad is the salad bar and the salad bar restaurant. Aside from a green salad and toppings, salad bar restaurants offer:

Macaroni salad (186 calories/serving), potato salad (107), tuna salad (383), and pasta salad (200). Then there is garlic bread (150 calories/slice), pizza (230+/slice), pasta (210), and soups (some of which are creamed or filled with pasta and cheese—200+). Of course, there is dessert like chocolate pudding cake (360) to be considered, and perhaps a glass of wine (120) or bottle of beer (150) with the meal.

You can fool yourself into feeling virtuous and yet cause yourself considerable damage. Adjusting for portion size, the box above weighs in at about 2300 calories, or 230 year-pounds. It will take about four and a third hours of high impact aerobics to burn this meal off. Is it worth it? Be sure before you eat. Maybe save some calories for another meal at another place.

Key 11: Beware of the vegetarian myth and the low fat fallacy.

It is important to understand the vegetarian myth and the low fat fallacy. Some people equate being a vegetarian with perfect health. Certainly, there are some important health advantages, but weight is not automatically one of them. As an example, a rhinoceros is totally vegan and weighs between four thousand and six thousand pounds. Healthy, but heavy.

Vegetarians tend to eat many carbohydrates. Carbohydrates have half the calories of fat, but carbohydrates do not turn off hunger pangs as readily as fats and proteins, so it is easier to over-eat carbohydrates. You can eat bowls and bowls of rice and still feel hungry. *Each cup of rice is about two hundred calories or twenty year-pounds.*

In place of meat, vegetarians often eat foods high in calories; cheese and milk products for instance. Soy products have the perception of being healthy, low cal items, but note that soymilk has about the same calories as cow's milk. A half cup of firm tofu is 185 calories, and a half cup of dry roasted soy nuts is 390 calories, almost 40 *year-pounds.* One cup of granola can run 598 calories, almost 60 *year-pounds.* A serving of black beans and rice can be 370 calories. (A regular cheeseburger is only 310 calories.) While I am not espousing eating burgers instead of vegetarian fare, I am stressing that you be aware of what you are eating based on fact, not assumptions.

How a vegetarian item is prepared can also greatly affect caloric content. One fried vegetarian Indian samosa, not a huge item on your plate, is 369 calories. I am not debating the health value of a vegetarian lifestyle, I am simply pointing out that vegetarian food should not automatically be considered low calorie. *Vegetarian items can be sources of significant calories.*

So, if being a vegetarian can have its problems, what about low fat foods as an aid to weight loss? Perhaps surprisingly, the obesity problem in the United States escalated in the 1980s commensurate with the rise of low fat food promotions by the food industry. Does this indicate we must eat more fat to lose weight? No. Let me explain.

All calories count. People tend to eat larger portions of low fat items because they have the misconception that they are also lower in calories. Not necessarily. Often low fat foods contain increased sugar and sweeteners to boost taste lost by lowering the fat content. These add calories. *Reduced fat peanut butter for instance, contains about the same calories as regular peanut butter.* In addition, sugars and carbohydrates stimulate the appetite, and carbohydrates do not satisfy your hunger as well as fats and proteins. Thus, unless you monitor your portion size carefully, it is easy to eat too much of a good thing. Even though carbohydrates are about half the calories of fat, eating too much of them can cause weight gain. Lower fat foods are better for your heart, but calories are calories in terms of your waist.

The approach, as always, is portion control and watching calories. Decide on a portion of food based on calories or *year-pounds*, not satiety, and you will do fine. If not, you may eat twice as many low fat cookies, and gain rather than lose weight. If you usually eat three cookies, do not eat six of the reduced fat (and hopefully reduced calorie) cookies. There are actually two ways to look at the concept of "light" foods. Take cream cheese as an example. If you like the taste of light cream cheese and eat a usual portion, you will benefit from the lower fat content. If you eat too much of it, you won't. *If, on the other hand, you only like the taste of regular cream cheese, you can make it "light" by eating less of it!* Perhaps not quite as good for your heart because of its higher fat content, but remember we are focusing on weight.

One way to improve satiety and avoid eating too many carbohydrates or low fat foods is to be sure you are getting adequate amounts of protein in your diet. Because you feel full after eating protein-rich foods, you tend to eat less and feel full sooner. The appetite satisfying effects of fat and protein are the basis of the high protein diets currently in vogue. However, these diets have health concerns in terms of cardiovascular disease, and these plans are monotonous and almost never followed for long periods. Studies have shown that high protein diets do not result in significant sustained weight loss.[13] Keep adequate, but not excessive amounts of protein in your diet. Continue to monitor calories and weight no matter what you are eating. Moderation is the key. Do not exclude any food group, but rather eat appropriate amounts of each. A skewed diet never works for long, no matter which way it points.

Key 12: Beware of fad diets.

What about the "other diets," and all the confusion that surrounds them? Frankly, all these diets call for fewer calories and more exercise. To be published and make it into the press, these diets are purposely more complex than they need to be. They all have a "hook." To attract the dieter's eye, they need to be trendy or ritualized. And as shown by a recent study in the *Journal of the American Medical Association*, these diets all have only limited efficacy because of lack of compliance.[14]

Two of my favorite examples of fad diets that have these hooks are the cabbage soup diet and the Atkins-type diet.

Years ago, the cabbage soup diet was in vogue based on the ritual of making your own cabbage soup and eating it regularly. After a while, you'd gradually introduce some protein in the form of chicken, etc. Boiled down (forgive the pun), the diet was composed of lots of water and vegetables—very low calorie items. In addition, it led to monotony and boredom. It worked in promoting weight reduction for a short period, but none of my patients were able to sustain this diet, and thus gained weight back, and often they gained additional pounds as well. The cabbage soup diet worked as a jump-start, but was impractical for prolonged dieting. This diet marketed packaging, not product. If I told patients to eat only vegetables and water for days on end, they would almost certainly balk. But, ask them to meticulously brew up some vegetable soup according to a very specific recipe, then they were all for it—even though it was only water and vegetables!

High protein, low carbohydrate diets are in vogue now. Volumes have been written about these diets—pro and con. Of particular note; however, is a review article on low carbohydrate diets in the *Journal of the American Medical Association* confirming weight loss on these diets was due simply to reduced caloric intake.[15] It all goes back to self-control and portion control. Nothing new—eat less, lose weight.

It is true that fat and protein turn off the appetite center better than sweets and carbohydrates (carbs). Fat and protein make you feel full so you automatically quit eating. Carbohydrates stimulate insulin release that lowers blood sugar and can result in a stimulus to eat more in an attempt to bring the blood sugar back up. Note, however, that carbohydrates are about half the calories of fat. So, if you do not respond to your appetite stimulus from carbs, but rather eat according to a plan, you can lose weight on a carbohydrate rich diet. High protein diets satisfy hunger, but are nutritionally unsound. A link exists between fats and heart problems, and the breakdown byproducts of fat and protein are difficult for the body to handle. Witness the fact that people with liver or kidney problems must limit their protein intake and eat more carbohydrates because metabolizing protein produces toxic byproducts that are difficult for the body to handle. One of these byproducts is ammonia. Have you ever smelled ammonia? Carbs are not all bad, and fat and protein are not the end-all. Above all, fad diets simply do not work over time as noted in the April 9, 2003 study in the *Journal of the American Medical Association*[13].

I could go on and on about diets and cite lots of literature, but in the end, you would spend a lot of time reading, and return to the same concept—total calorie intake and exercise govern weight loss or gain. So let's keep it short and sweet. Spend time doing, not deliberating. Don't look for the magic diet or pill. None exists. Losing weight is straightforward, if done in gradual steps. Start today. Save your time and money looking for the quick fix diet. The answer to weight loss is within your grasp. Leave a hundred and twenty calories a day or a quarter pound a week on the table.

 ## Key 13: Beware of restaurants.

Restaurants, like spices, are to be enjoyed in small quantities. Like spices, restaurants can enhance the flavor of your life. Taken to excess, they can lead to losing control of your weight loss program; just as too many spices can ruin a good dish. As I have said previously, I urge you to occasionally go to a restaurant, relax, and enjoy yourself. Without breaks from your routine, you will not be able to sustain your weight loss program. Remember, losing weight has to be enjoyable.

It is nearly impossible to eat carefully in a restaurant, but you can at least practice damage control. And this is all I ask on your occasional outings.

The purpose of a restaurant is to serve food that is unique and tasty. Health is not generally an issue; having you return to dine again, is. Unfortunately, most palates appreciate fat, salt, and sugar, which is why restaurant food tends to be high in these items. *Even if you think you are eating healthfully, you may not be since you have little control over what goes on in the restaurant's kitchen.*

Let me give you two examples from my experiences. The first is for those of you who order fish instead of meats or poultry. I was speaking to a chef who was a patient of mine, and she told me she used a half stick of butter when she prepared a piece of fish (415 calories for butter alone, that's 41.5 *year-pounds*). Even if much of the butter just ends up on the plate after you've eaten the fish, a lot of the butter still mixes in with the vegetables and other foods (which may have their own sauces in addition). Okay, so you are smart and order your fish grilled with herbs and no butter or oil except a blush of olive oil to hold the condiments. You avoid the butter trap.

Now, let's move on to the salad. Here again I have an anecdote that makes a point about lack of control over what you eat in a restaurant. My wife and I frequented a particular restaurant many times, and she always ordered a Caesar salad. I opted for a simple green salad with honey mustard vinaigrette, which I assumed was healthier and less caloric. My choice seemed so virtuous. When salmonella became a problem in raw eggs, my wife asked the server one day how the chef continued to make a Caesar dressing without fresh eggs. The server said the chef used a pasteurized egg yolk product instead of raw eggs. The server also added that the chef used the egg yolk product in *all* of the salad dressings to add consistency and flavor—even the honey mustard vinaigrette. What I thought was low cholesterol, low calorie dressing was in fact, neither.

Different restaurant cuisines can affect your calorie count. Mexican and Chinese foods tend to have more fat and calories than Japanese or Italian. This, of course, depends on what you order, but you have a better chance of this excess in certain cuisine. Also, remember the vegetarian myth. For example, Indian vegetarian dishes can contain high calorie items like coconut milk and cheese. Similarly, Chinese vegetable dishes might contain a lot of oil. And don't overlook the problems of deadly salads discussed earlier and in Key 10.

A salad of greens and fresh vegetables with a light dressing or just lemon juice or balsamic vinegar can be a wonderful thing. What happens next—often at a salad bar—can turn the tide toward a high calorie item. Dressings, nuts, cheeses, croutons, and bacon bits, etcetera, can quickly add up to a high calorie meal. If you add pasta, muffins, and a dessert often offered at salad bar restaurants, you're on your way—the wrong way. You pride yourself that you are having a salad instead of "a meal," but in fact, you may have packed away more calories than a simple dinner. I am not saying don't eat salads or don't go to a salad bar.

Just apply your usual principles of portion control, noting calories, and deciding if all the toppings and other items are "to die for."

Unless you investigate the preparation of each food item ordered and make modifications (not always possible), you are at the mercy of the chef. If you make too many changes in your food order, you'll end up with fairly tasteless food. A friend of mine used to order steamed vegetables and rice when he went to a Chinese restaurant ... pretty bland stuff he could have made at home. I doubt such food would satisfy cravings during a weekly restaurant outing.

So what do you do about the restaurant dilemma?

One cannot sustain an unwavering weight loss regimen. You need some time off. Once a week, if you have done well with your weight program, go out for dinner. Splurge a little ... *a little.* Enjoy yourself, but practice portion control. Order smaller portions if they are offered. Share an entrée, appetizer, or dessert. Order salad dressing on the side or simply use balsamic vinegar or lemon juice. Watch the amount of bread and butter you eat, and if the bread is really good, you should be able to enjoy it without butter. Consider having a mineral water or iced tea instead of alcohol, or at least order wine by the glass, not by the bottle.

If a particularly high calorie item catches your eye, ask yourself, "Is it really to die for?" If not, consider ordering a lower calorie item. If it is really "to die for," order and enjoy, that's why you are dining out. You will not gain five pounds from one meal! It's the repeated offenses that add up to a problem. Excess calories consumed over and over again are the issue. So, while you may gain a little weight from one indiscretion, you will have enjoyed yourself and be willing during the following week to find a few extra ounces to discard in order to compensate. You have a whole week to make up for modest indiscretions, but the word is "modest." Similarly, eating out too frequently or bringing home takeout food too often will add up, get ahead of you, and put you on the slippery slope to weight gain and failure.

Some real life choices while dining out.

Let's say you and your significant other go out to dinner at a new restaurant, Café Lido, a quaint little family run establishment. You look over the menu carefully. Instead of the Brie, you decide on a smoked salmon appetizer. You save 217 calories. On your mixed greens salad you use one or two tablespoons of Italian dressing instead of double what the chef might be using. You save another 86 calories. You split the filet mignon. (Notice I'm not even insisting on fish or chicken.) Add another 100 calories to your savings account. You choose a baked potato with butter if you like, instead of au gratin potatoes, saving an additional 177 calories—unless you insist on sour cream and chives then you save only 117 calories. You order steamed asparagus, asking the chef to hold the gobs of butter he uses, adding it yourself if you must, but in a controlled manner. Next, on to dessert—apple pie—your favorite. You've been good and you've heard the pie here is *to die for*, so you order the dessert with anticipation. When the pie arrives at the table, you notice it's à la mode. As we discussed before, you wanted the pie and were willing to deal with the calories, but had not counted on it being à la mode. So push the ice cream aside, and enjoy the pie to its fullest. That's really what you ordered anyway. This would most likely save you 150 to 250 calories. *Including dessert, the above decisions saved you about 720 calories, or 72 year-pounds. You had a wonderful meal and a great time, and saved yourself one and three-quarters hours exercising on a treadmill to burn off the extra calories you would have eaten, had you not made these changes.*

In terms of controlling calories, you are the best chef because you can watch each ingredient and control how your food is prepared. Eating at home most of the week is best. But with a little care and a few wise choices, you can enjoy food prepared by Chef So-and-So, have a great evening dining out with friends, and feel ready to continue with your weight management program the following morning.

 Key 14: Be a food snob.

Perhaps this is a good time to introduce the concept of being a food snob. *This is a positive term, not a negative one. A food snob is a person who refuses to waste calories on any food that is not "to die for." The flip side is that this person is wildly happy and satisfied because he or she enjoys wonderful food and drink. I am convinced you will lose weight and keep it off only if the process of weight loss is not intrusive and your eating experiences are pleasurable.* The process needs to be rewarding. You cannot give up everything you love to eat and get nothing in return except weight loss. Some diets insist on no pasta, no bread, no "white foods," no sweets, no variety, no to almost everything. Any weight loss that occurs is often due to boredom and taste fatigue. You just can't sustain a very limited diet forever. *Remember, weight management is forever; not just*

the length of time you can eat a prescribed set of foods. Most people need more fun and excitement in their lives than losing weight by giving up all the foods they like.

Let me give you some examples of how to be a food snob, and love it! Let's say you're at a wedding reception and they are serving inexpensive wine and those prefabricated hors d'oeuvres that all taste about the same even though they look different. And, of course, there is the standard wedding cake. Many people overeat just because they are there and the food is available. *Two glasses of wine, three to four canapés and a piece of wedding cake would be about seven hundred calories (seventy year-pounds, or the weight of fourteen bags of flour on a yearly basis). Is it worth it?*

If you were a food snob, you would assess the situation and have a mineral water, some vegetables and bread, and pass on the cake completely. To be a bit festive, you might indulge in a martini (175 calories) or a glass of scotch (90 calories) rather than the mediocre wine. The calories will still count, but be enjoyable. No calories wasted, less time on the treadmill. How then can you not be happy? With the calories saved, you can go out afterward to a favorite restaurant and have an excellent meal using some of the saved calories. Or, you could have eaten some wonderful, favorite foods at home before the event and eat only for "social reasons," not wanting to appear impolite. The calories saved can be put in the bank to be used in the future. If later on you are attending another event where the food and drink are "to die for," go for it. Indulge. Have seconds if you like. You have calories in the bank from previous social events.

By being a food snob you are not denying yourself pleasure, you are simply deferring it. By eating on your own terms, you can be even happier. You will constantly be treating yourself to the best foods and drink, not wasting calories on the mediocre stuff. This even works out economically. Let's say you drink one glass of wine a day, and the bottle costs $10. If instead, you drank a glass every three days, you could afford a $30 bottle of wine and save calories at the same time. Better wine, fewer calories. If you are worried about spoilage, don't be. There is an inexpensive, easy to use, inert gas wine preservative available in most liquor stores and in many cooking stores. If you do not want to use the preservative, you could opt to buy a half bottle of wine or share a bottle with friends once or twice a week. Instead of eating a large chunk of generic cheddar cheese, have a smaller amount of a wonderful specialty cheese. Fewer calories, more enjoyment. Pamper yourself. Eat better quality foods, and lose weight without feeling deprived.

 Key 15: Enlist others in your quest.

Why be a food snob alone? Part of enjoying food is the social experience. Part of losing weight is the support of others. Enlisting others in your quest makes the journey easier and more fun.

It's very difficult to stop smoking if someone around you continues to smoke. Similarly, it is difficult to work on weight loss if someone who eats with you is bent on eating as many calories as possible. How then can you enlist this person's help? The answer is by example.

At this point, you are hopefully enjoying losing weight and happy in your role as a food snob. Communicating this to your culinary partner by your actions is a first step. If he or she sees you are happy while losing weight, chances are your partner will be willing to go along with dietary changes. If you were on a diet that made you unhappy and you were constantly complaining, things would be different. Initially you may have to "do your thing" alone, but if you stick to your new eating habits and are happy about it, the chances are your partner will come around. Then both of you can work together, and in time a lot of the edible temptations will disappear from the house, making it even easier to stay on your program … together.

If you are not able to enlist your partner in your quest, so be it. Remember, you are happy with your weight loss program as you have structured it, and you will simply continue.

What about dining with friends in their homes? Do you need to inform them you are working on your weight so they prepare foods differently when you visit? This is up to you. It would be considerate, but remember you can lose weight by eating regular food, just less of it. You may choose to tell your friends, or you can simply self-regulate. You do not need to be in the spotlight or feel you are inconveniencing them by asking for special foods. Instead of, "Sandy, I'm on a diet. Please don't have starch with dinner." You can simply ask for just a "taste" of the potatoes and leave the bread in the basket. When your friends notice your weight loss and ask how you did it, you can explain. They may be interested in changing their eating habits thanks to your success.

Key 16: Exercise is a must, but easier than you think.

Many books have been written about exercise, and I am not going to reiterate what is already in print. I want to simply set forth some general principles as in other chapters.

Exercise is important in accelerating a weight loss program. It is additive to calorie reduction. *If in addition to cutting out a hundred and twenty calories a day, you burn off the same amount exercising, you will lose weight twice as fast—twenty-four pounds in a year.* To burn a hundred and twenty calories requires little exercise. A leisurely ten mile per hour bike ride for thirty minutes will do the trick.

Exercise is important to help maintain a weight loss program. As you lose weight, your metabolism slows down and it becomes harder to lose weight. This actually makes sense.

Let's say you were an animal in the forest and food is scarce in the winter. You would begin to lose weight as the result of decreased caloric intake. This could be a problem if weight loss continued and you lost too much weight before the grasses and berries returned in the spring. As a result, as you lose weight, your metabolism slows so you can survive the winter on less food. A hibernating bear is good example.

Even when we lose weight by choice, our metabolism slows despite a full refrigerator. We want to continue to lose weight despite a slower adaptive metabolism. We need to force the body to burn more calories even as we lose weight. How? Exercise. Exercise burns calories regardless of weight, and independently of what your body's calorie thermostat dictates. Exercise is very important in sustaining weight loss and minimizing plateaus, a problem often referred to as "hitting the wall."

How much exercise do you need? My answer? Enough. My approach to exercise is similar to that of calories. There are guidelines, but they are for the population at large, not for you as an individual. I suggest you simply begin by doing a bit more than you are now. If you are not exercising at all, begin by a brief walk, a short bicycle ride, even just five minutes on a treadmill. You need to start somewhere and you want your goal to be attainable. Remember, if you are not currently exercising, a little workout is a one hundred percent increase. If you are already exercising regularly, simply kick it up a bit. *Twelve minutes more, five times a week, is an extra hour a week of exercise. That's more than fifty hours per year.* You should not overdo your exercise routine or do too much too soon. Small, regular incremental increases work well. *Just like taking weight loss an ounce at a time, take exercise a step at a time. The steps will add up just as the ounces do. Nickels and dimes add up to dollars.*

I like to think of two types of exercise, formal and informal. Both are important. Examples of formal exercise are running, swimming, bicycling, attending aerobic classes, working out at the gym, etc. Informal exercise takes place during everyday life; simply getting through your day constitutes exercise. Walking around, climbing stairs, gardening, stacking firewood, shopping, and walking to the refrigerator for food expend calories. Even chewing your food burns eleven calories per hour, though I caution you about eating *more* to increase your caloric burn! And, there is no way you can chew enough sugarless gum to burn off a crème brulée.

▶ *Formal Exercise*

Just as there is a difference between eating for your heart or your weight, there is a difference between exercising for your heart and exercising to lose weight. General teaching is that exercising twenty minutes, three times a week at your target heart rate, promotes cardiac fitness and increases your high-density lipoprotein, or good cholesterol. This is very important and I urge this be part of your exercise program. But for weight loss, I recommend you exercise an additional two to three times a week. Even if it's not as vigorous a program as the other three days, the extra workout is still beneficial. Remember, each one hundred calories burned is ten pounds a year. *Lower intensity exercise below your target heart rate may not directly benefit the heart as much, but the resulting weight loss benefits the heart indirectly.* Commensurate with this, as of 2006, the American Heart Association is now recommending thirty minutes of daily activity at some level in order to help with weight control.

Formal exercise, done correctly, is by nature more demanding on the body than informal exercise. Don't overdo it. When you begin your program start slowly. You have plenty of time to build up your exercise program. You don't need to do it in one week. Take jogging as an example. Begin by walking a short distance, then increase the distance as is comfortable. When this seems routine, you can begin jogging, gradually picking up speed and duration. *Listen to your body. Do not push too hard or too fast. If you injure yourself by overdoing, you will need to stop exercising for a while, and then you will have to begin all over again. That's why I use the phrase, "Exercise less to exercise more."*

As you get older, you will need to lower your exercise goals commensurate with aging. In your youthful exuberance, you can run aggressively, injure your knees, and have to give up jogging. Or you can be temperate in your program and exercise for years and years. As an example, I have jogged for thirty years. I used to jog six miles a day four to five times a week. I am still jogging, but now for only two to three miles, five times a week and at a slower pace. I no longer jog competitively. I have had no injuries to date because I've lowered the intensity of my jogging program, and I look forward to many more years of this exercise. Friends who didn't listen to their naturally aging bodies are no longer jogging. Exercise less to exercise more. *By tempering your exercise and not overdoing it, chances are you will be able to exercise years longer and come out ahead. Slow and steady wins the race. This principle holds true for exercise as it does for weight loss.*

How hard do I need to exercise for benefit? Any level of exercise is better than none at all. A more exact way to determine an appropriate level of exercise is to use your target heart rate. You can obtain this number by taking a treadmill exam at your physician's office. There are also tables and formulas that give an approximation without the expense of a treadmill test. The Web site *www. dummies.com* has a page on how to determine your target heart rate. Twenty minutes of exercise in your target heart rate zone, three times a week, will keep your heart healthy. Allow a five to ten minute warm up and cool down period to prevent injury and cardiac problems. And remember, your weight program will benefit from even more frequent exercise, even at a lower intensity, be it formal or informal.

Frequency of exercise, if not excessive, also has other benefits. Make exercise a part of your daily routine. The longer you exercise regularly, the easier it becomes. By this, I mean the exercise program becomes a part of your day and you feel uncomfortable if you don't exercise. It becomes a habit, in the good sense. Make exercise a priority. Given the demands of daily life, if you fit exercise into your schedule *only* when all else is completed, you will rarely exercise. Better to set a regular time to exercise and commit to it. Inform those around you of your commitment to that time slot, and you will be more successful. Each morning I choose 5:30 to exercise, before the demands of the day begin. This may not be practical for you, but almost everyone has some time in the day to spare. *Remember, weight loss responds to even low levels of regular exercise. As little as ten minutes of exercise a day adds up to more than an hour a week.* This is not adequate for the heart (though better than no exercise), but definitely helps with weight loss. Nickels and dimes do add up.

Exercising on a regular basis keeps the body in shape for even more exercising. Aggressive workouts only on weekends (the "weekend warrior"), stresses the body's joints and tendons because they are not regularly stretched. This is a potential problem. Regular exercise helps prevent injuries.

Along the lines of preventing injury, I cannot stress enough the need to change your exercise shoes regularly. Shoes continue to look good on the outside long after they have ceased to function in terms of support, cushioning, and protecting the feet. A good rule of thumb is to change your shoes every three hundred and fifty to five hundred miles that you've run or walked.

A step at a time, just fine. As noted earlier, I am a great proponent of exercise on a regular basis. However, many people do not keep up with an exercise program anymore than they do with a fad diet. This is because the diet or the exercise program is intrusive and therefore eventually falls by the wayside. The level of effort and commitment is simply more than the individual will put forth. This is why I propose a subliminal approach to weight loss—an ounce at a time. I suggest this approach works for exercise as well. Exercise a step at a time. An exercise program needs to be as seamless as possible, and work within the parameters of your lifestyle. One way is to make formal exercise less formidable. Another is to use the benefits of informal exercise.

"Exercise less to exercise more." *Hour-long workouts at the gym are fine if you have the time and are into them. But there is also travel time to and from the gym, and membership dues to consider. This is a large commitment and may lead to failure. Remember, set attainable goals, and reach them over and over.* Let's take each aspect separately.

Any exercise is better than none. If you don't have the time on occasion (or maybe several occasions) for your full workout, do a shorter one. Don't feel guilty or say, "Since I don't have time for a complete workout, I won't do any today." Commonly, today then becomes tomorrow and the next day, and when the regularity and momentum are broken, failure to exercise at all looms on the horizon.

This leads into my next issue—*the drive to the gym. I believe that this drive is often a barrier to success. Even if it's only a ten minute drive each way that's one hour a week if you work out three times. If it's a fifteen minute drive, that's one and a half hours per week. A half-hour trip each way three times a week is three hours, almost half a workday. This is time sitting that you could have spent exercising (or doing something else). Also, don't forget the time you might spend at the gym waiting for a piece of equipment to become available.* What is the solution? Have a backup program!

I suggest you have exercise equipment to use at home when you don't feel like going to the gym, or have only limited time. This will allow you to use your time exercising rather than sitting in the car. Having exercise equipment at home will prevent you from having to drive in inclement weather conditions that might make the trek to the gym less than fun.

My favorite piece of home exercise equipment is a treadmill. The newer ones are inexpensive (they cost less than most gym memberships) and come in relatively compact sizes if you avoid all the extra bells and whistles found on the larger units.

No space for a treadmill? Then how about a stationary bicycle or stair stepper? Select a piece of exercise equipment that you find easy to use, and be willing to use it occasionally, if not every day. Some equipment requires learning a new set of skills. Many of my patients bought a NordicTrack, but after a while, the equipment ended up as an expensive clothes rack. While NordicTrack provides excellent exercise, you don't simply hop on and begin, it takes practice. This is why I like the treadmill. *Everyone who can walk can use a treadmill.* You can jog, run, and climb hills on a treadmill, using skills most of us already possess. Is the treadmill the best exercise program? Rather than get into this debate, I would maintain *any exercise program you do regularly is the best program.* In the dark of night, or when the weather is rainy or snowy, your treadmill is there in a safe, private, and cozy environment for you to use. No time wasted traveling to and from the gym. No need to dress up, comb your hair or brush your teeth, you've "ordered in" exercise. No one will see you or judge you.

Let me give you a scenario. You get home at five o'clock and you'd like to exercise, but you have dinner reservations at seven. No time to go to the gym, which would take at least an hour and a half including travel time. But you could get on your treadmill for fifteen minutes, warm up, cool down, shower, and still make the dinner reservation. Not a long exercise program, but better than none, and no travel time required.

Another aspect of a treadmill I like is that it is a natural extension of your daily routine: walking or jogging. Thus, when you go on a trip, all the exercise equipment you need to bring with you are your workout shoes. If your hotel doesn't have a gym you can always walk, jog, run or "do the stairs" at the hotel utilizing the same muscles and principles you use at home. This prevents disruption of your regular program, which is very important.

▶ Informal Exercise

This is my favorite type of exercise because it fits best with my ounce at a time, step at a time approach to weight loss. *Yes, you will definitely benefit from a formal exercise program, but this takes a level of commitment that some of you might not have. Just like looking for small calorie changes in your diet instead of massive ones, look for little ways to increase your exercise and caloric expenditure. The trick is to exercise repeatedly, so the calories burned add up to ounces and then pounds.*

Exercise adds up just as calories do. Take the stairs instead of the elevator. Even if your office is on the thirtieth floor and you can't walk all the way, walk several flights, and then take the elevator. Park a distance away from a store and walk to it rather than seek out the nearest parking spot. Nothing is more amusing than watching people jockey for the closest parking spots when they are going to the gym to exercise.

I put a small water glass on my desk at work necessitating my getting up frequently for refills. I also bring only a few patient charts at a time to the filing area, so I have to make several trips. I could make it in one trip, but I use the several scattered trips as a brief workout break. *Every three steps you take burn about one calorie, so as little as three hundred and sixty steps give you your one hundred and twenty calories for the day.*

Look for little ways to exercise in everything you do. Walking in place while you brush your teeth burns calories. Tapping your feet while sitting at your desk talking on the phone also counts. And, how about walking down the hall to talk to someone instead of phoning, messaging, or e-mailing? These may not be aerobic or cardiovascular, but they burn calories. If you think as much as you can about keeping in motion, you will come up with many ideas of your own. These are the nickels and dimes of exercise, the small change under the sofa cushions.

In summary, make a commitment to exercise regularly, even if your life permits only short workouts. Make exercise fun and a part of your life, not an intrusion. Do what works for you, be it going to the gym, exercising at home, hiring a personal trainer, jogging, walking, etc. Exercise carefully to avoid injury. Change your exercise shoes regularly. Get exercise instruction when needed. Build a repertoire of informal daily exercises that are actually part of your usual routine. View exercise in blocks of minutes not hours, and in time these blocks will add up to hours.

 Key 17: Break the rules.

If you're going to stay on your weight management program for life, you need to enjoy your program or you will fail. Remember, you design the agenda. Nothing is imposed. You can modify and change the rules at any time as long as you follow the few basic principles. You decide how fast to lose the weight. You decide how many calories to eat and when. The only requirement is that you maintain a gradual weight loss. If you are not enjoying the weight management program, it's not because of imposed rules. Change your approach. You have a barometer of success, the scale. If you are happy and your weight is decreasing at any speed, you are succeeding. Work with the principles. You can change them to meet your needs as long as you are winning. Do what works for you.

After reading my original manuscript, one of my friends told me he found the small calorie approach to weight loss quite helpful. He liked to eat and was not into dieting, but wanted to lose weight. He was willing to make some small changes in his eating habits, so he came up with a simple idea that worked well for him. Every day at lunch he drank a regular cola. He did not like the taste of diet cola, but wanted something more exciting than water. He came to realize a regular cola contained many calories, but rather than give up and switch to diet cola, he found an easy solution. He simply reversed how he filled his glass. He used to fill the glass with cola from a large bottle and then add the ice cubes, now he fills his glass full of ice first, then pours in the cola. This method cut down on the amount of cola (and calories) he consumed, and he maintained that the cola was colder and actually tasted better. A win-win situation. A simple step he was willing and proud to take as a first step toward weight management.

I wrote earlier about eating more to eat less. By this I meant that skipping meals could lead to increased appetite and difficulty regulating how much you eat when you do eat. But for some people this is not a problem. They can go all day without eating, feel good, and still eat reasonably at dinner. Similarly, some people do better with a big breakfast or lunch and a small dinner, which is the opposite of what most Americans tend toward. If this works, do it. You may occasionally want just pie for breakfast, or cheese and crackers for dinner. If it works for you and reduces calories at the end of the day, it's okay. Overall, the idea is to eat healthily, but not necessarily all the time. Remember, if you are on the quarter pound program, you are no doubt well ahead of your earlier eating habits, so an occasional slip is okay. We are focusing on weight loss, not total health consciousness at each meal. One thing at a time. We learn to read by starting with words, not sentences. So, at first, we're simply focusing on ounces. Our goal is to lose an ounce at a time, not a pound at a time. Once we get the general principles of weight loss under our belt (forgive the pun), we can add additional concepts about fats, food balance, etc. *Keep dieting simple and lose weight. Flood your mind with too many rules and formulas and you will fail. Remember, this is a simple approach to weight loss for people who prefer to do things other than focus on diet.*

There are very few do's and don'ts to my approach. Do what works. You are in control, not being controlled. In time, as you are more and more successful and the weight management process becomes second nature, it will become easier to add a few more rules about nutrition that can make your approach even healthier.

The seeming contradiction here is that as you think more about your weight, you will think less about your weight. By this I mean that as you adopt the quarter pound approach and lose weight by discarding small calories, a bite at a time, you will not constantly be preoccupied with your weight. Yes, you will always need to look for calories to shave off, but you will not have to focus on your weight per se because you will be losing subliminally.

You won't be lusting over foods you cannot have because you can have them—if you want to—though hopefully in a smaller portion than in the past. And since your weight is down, gaining a pound or two on occasion will not put you into an emotional tailspin. You will simply have to look for some "spare change under the sofa cushions," some additional calories to shave off. The focus is on the calories and *year-pounds*, not your reflection in the mirror.

IN CONCLUSION

WRITE YOUR OWN BOOK

If you have read this book, you now understand my "Truisms and Seeming Contradictions."

- ➢ TO LOSE WEIGHT, DON'T DIET
- ➢ SLOW WEIGHT LOSS IS FASTER THAN FAST WEIGHT LOSS
- ➢ CHANGE LITTLE THINGS TO CHANGE A LOT
- ➢ ONE HUNDRED CALORIES A DAY EQUALS TEN POUNDS A YEAR
- ➢ EAT MORE TO EAT LESS
- ➢ EXERCISE LESS TO EXERCISE MORE
- ➢ COOK MORE TO COOK LESS
- ➢ THE FREEZER IS YOUR FRIEND; RESTAURANTS ARE NOT

You now understand the power of the ounce, and that weight is lost one bite at a time. You recognize how everyday tasks such as climbing stairs instead of taking the elevator can add significantly to your total daily exercise. You appreciate that small, repetitive food and lifestyle changes have a profound influence on weight loss. In addition, you understand it's possible to lose weight successfully, enjoy eating, and have a life. Above all, you know you can now succeed even if you've failed before.

I have given you very few rules, or do's and don'ts about managing your weight, and even these are open to interpretation. Try different things to see what works for you, and what you find successful. Maybe dessert before dinner? No one knows you as well as you. Let the scale be your guide as to whether you are succeeding in attaining your weight goal. When it comes to weight loss, no one is an expert or has all the answers. Each of us is different. So, within the general principles outlined in this book, experiment. Add your own ideas. Write your own book, figuratively or literally.

As a physician, I always tell my patients that medicine is a team sport. A good doctor enlists the help of his patient and they work together on health matters. Similarly, I feel that weight problems need to be worked on together. This book is my contribution to that goal. I hope it will inspire you to lose weight by demonstrating how easy weight loss can be, even if difficult in the past. The power is within you. Keep your eye on the ounces and the pounds will follow.

APPENDIX I

CALORIES AND *YEAR-POUNDS*

The pages that follow are a brief summary of calories contained in a variety of common foods. While not intended to be comprehensive, the list illustrates examples of how to trim away calories and find those four ounces. Values are approximations based on portion size, though the portion sizes used are often small by today's standards of "super-sizing." Therefore, the values are often underestimated, and some values are averaged. As stated in the text, the same item made by different manufacturers could vary considerably in terms of calorie content. Therefore, I suggest you use the chart not as an absolute, but as a general guide to choosing among the various options. Don't worry if the apple you are eating is seventy or eighty-five calories, but rather that on average, you can have a grapefruit for less. It is the relative values, not the absolutes that are important.

I call your attention to the *year-pounds* column, calculated by dividing calories by ten. This is the weight attributed to eating the item every day for a year. If that happens to exceed the calories per day that you need to maintain your weight, this will then represent the amount of weight you will gain eating this food on a daily basis. A small one hundred calorie item eaten daily represents ten *year-pounds*. Many of us don't understand calories. Are one hundred calories a little or a lot? We might not know calories, but we know pounds. Ten pounds is two, five-pound bags of sugar! We know how that feels in our grocery bag, and on our beltline.

There is no need to memorize the appendix. Simply review it to grasp the big picture. Find some choices that will allow you to discard those daily hundred and twenty calories, your four ounces a week.

Try switching to nonfat milk, or have a half grapefruit instead of a glass of orange juice. I think you'll find the chart easy to use and helpful, though again, not inclusive. I am not singling out any particular manufacturer or fast food restaurant; I am simply giving some examples to stimulate your thinking. Items may not be completely comparable. For instance, a simple garden salad has fewer ingredients than a mandarin chicken salad, and obviously has fewer calories. This is not a revelation, and this is not to say you shouldn't eat the mandarin chicken salad if you want to; it is simply to show the difference so you can make an informed choice rather than assume all salads are a calorie bargain.

You may want to know the calories or *year-pounds* of foods beyond the scope of this list. The calorie content of foods is available from many sources. There are numerous books published that list the nutritional content of foods. There are many Web sites on the Internet that list similar information. In fact, the department of agriculture has an extensive list of food values at *www.usda.gov*. You can also do a Google search for a specific food item by entering "Calories in...."

Have fun playing the game "How Low Can I Go?" How many calories (*year-pounds*) can I shave off and still thoroughly enjoy my food, my life, and the fact that I am losing weight easily and permanently?

A Brief and Informative Food Comparison Chart

Food	Calories	Year-Pounds (Approximate)	Simple Numbers to Remember and Points of Note
BREAKFAST			
Juices & Fruit Apple or Orange juice	111	11	*Summary:*
▶1 Orange	65	6.5	Figure juices at about 110 cal. But note:
▶1 Apple	81	8.1	▶A piece of fruit is 30–50 fewer calories
Grapefruit juice	96	9.6	*Hi cal. juices:*
▶½ Grapefruit	37	3.7	▶nectars 150
Tomato juice	32	3.2	▶prune juice 180
Prune juice	181	18.1	*Lo cal.* ▶tomato 30 (but high in salt)
Cereals Cold cereal ¾–1 cup	90–110	10	*Summary:*
▶National brand sweetened bran cereal per ⅓ cup	108 (=324 *per cup*)	10.8/32.4	Figure average cereal at about 110 cal. However, note that some cereals and granola are considerably higher. (▶Note serving size.)
Hot cereal (plain) ¾ cup	100–115	10–11.5	
▶Flavored like cinnamon & spice	177	17.7	Remember:
▶Granola ¼ cup	130	13	▶You add calories for milk, sugar, and fruit if used.
			▶Note extra calories added by fruit … about 100–150 calories.
With sugar add …	15/tsp.	1.5	▶Note significant difference using nonfat milk.
With milk add …			
Whole	150/cup	15	
2 percent	120	12	
1 percent	100	10	
Nonfat	85	8.5	
With fruit add …			
Banana	105	10.5	
Dates ¼ cup	130	13	
Raisins ⅓ cup	150	15	
Dried figs 3	160	16	

	Food	Calories	Year-Pounds (Approximate)	Simple Numbers to Remember and Points of Note
Breads	Toast 1 slice	70	7	*Summary:*
	With butter add …	36/tsp.	3.6	These items add 150 to over 400 calories very quickly.
	With jam add …	52/Tbsp.	5.2	>> **Be Careful** <<
	With honey add …	65/Tbsp.	6.5	
	English, blueberry, or corn muffin	135	13.5	
	▶ Nat'l chain blueberry scone	460	46	
	Bagel	163–370	16.3–37	
	Bagel with 2 Tbsp. cream cheese	262–469	26.2–46.9	
	Bagel with 2 Tbsp. *Light cream cheese*	225–432	22.5–43.2	
	Banana nut muffin	371	37.1	
	Date nut muffin	427	42.7	
	Doughnut, glazed	230–310	23–31	
	Pancake each	70	7	
	With syrup add …	100/oz.	10	
	▶ *With light syrup add …*	55	5.5	
	With butter add …	36/tsp.	3.6	
	French toast each	70–95	7–9.5	
	With syrup add …	100/oz.	10	
	▶ *With light syrup add …*	55	5.5	
	With butter add …	36/tsp.	3.6	
Eggs, etc.	Egg boiled or poached, each	79	7.9	*Summary:*
	▶ Scrambled, each	95	9.5	Eggs are a pretty good deal. What you do with them is the issue.
	▶ Egg substitute	25	2.5	
	Western omelet	207	20.7	
	Cheddar cheese omelet	313	31.3	
	▶ Eggs Benedict	410	41	
	▶ Eggs Florentine	520	52	
	Add a side dish:			
	Bacon add …	36/slice	3.6	
	Sausage patty add …	100	10	
	Ham slice (3.5 oz) add …	203	20.3	
	▶ Fast food chain English muffin with egg, cheese, and ham	300	30	
	▶ As above, but with sausage instead	380	38	

	Food	Calories	Year-Pounds (Approximate)	Simple Numbers to Remember and Points of Note
Beverages	Coffee or Tea, Black	2–4	0.3	*Summary:*
	With sugar add ...	15/tsp.	1.5	Coffee and tea are almost free. What you do to them is another matter.
	With milk or cream			
	Cream add ...	37/Tbsp.	3.7	
	Half & half add ...	20	2	
	▶ Fat free half & half add ...	10	1	
	Whole milk add ...	9	0.9	
	2 percent milk add ...	7.5	0.75	
	1 percent milk add ...	6	0.6	
	▶ Nonfat milk add	5	0.5	
	▶ Non-dairy creamer	20	2	
	▶ *Nonfat creamer*	10	1	
	National chain café lattes			
	Small	200	20	
	Medium	260	26	
	Large	340	34	
	National chain nonfat café lattes			
	Small	120	12	
	Medium	160	16	
	Large	210	21	

LUNCH

	Food	Calories	Year-Pounds (Approximate)	Simple Numbers to Remember and Points of Note
Soups	Bouillon	5	0.5	*Summary:*
	Chicken noodle	75	7.5	Soup's a good deal. >But cream, beans, peas, lentils, etc., have more calories than a more basic soup like chicken noodle..
	Cream of chicken	117	11.7	
	Minestrone	96	9.6	
	Black bean	116	11.6	
	Lentil or split pea	140	14	
Salads	Dinner salad of greens & vegetables, no dressing	89	8.9	
				Summary:
				Salads can vary a lot depending what's in them and on them.
	With dressing:			
	Regular ranch *add ...*	148/2Tbsp.	14.8	
	▶ Fat free ranch *add ...*	48	4.8	
	With croutons add ...	122/cup	12.2	▼ continued next page

	Food	Calories	Year-Pounds (Approximate)	Simple Numbers to Remember and Points of Note
	With a topping like:			
	Seasoned almonds add ...	40/Tbsp.	4	
	▶ National chain mandarin style chicken salad	730	73	
	▶ National chain mixed green salad (with dressing & toppings)	690	69	
Sandwiches	▶ National chain turkey deli	215	21.5	*Summary:*
	National chain beef deli	223	22.3	Sandwich calories vary a lot. Consider making your own using low calorie items.
	▶ National chain tuna deli	325	32.5	
	▶ Nat'l chain hot beef and Swiss	810	81	
	Nat'l chain hot turkey and Swiss	760	76	
Fast Food Examples	*Hamburger chain*			*Summary:*
	Hamburger	260	26	*Fast Food Calories Add Up Fast ...*
	Cheeseburger	310	31	▶ Beans, salad, and fish are not always a calorie bargain.
	Deluxe large cheeseburger	560	56	
	▶ Deluxe double cheeseburger	730	73	
	Fried fish sandwich	400	40	
	French fries			
	Small	230	23	
	Medium	350	35	
	▶ Large	520	52	
	Mexican food chain			
	Soft beef taco	190	19	
	Soft chicken taco	170	17	
	Bean burrito	350	35	
	Beef burrito	440	44	
	Nachos	460	46	
	▶ Taco salad	610	61	
	Pizza chain			
	Personal size (the small one!)			
	Cheese	580	58	
	Pepperoni	640	64	
	▶ All meat pan style	1010	101	

	Food	Calories	Year-Pounds (Approximate)	Simple Numbers to Remember and Points of Note
Beverages	Soft drink	140	14	*Summary:*
				Diet drinks are a bargain if you like them.
	Diet soft drink	0	0	
	Iced tea, no sugar	0	0	
	With sugar add ...	15/tsp.	1.5	
	Milkshake	375	37.5	

DINNER

	Food	Calories	Year-Pounds (Approximate)	Simple Numbers to Remember and Points of Note
Cocktails	Small glass of wine (2 oz.)	72	7.2	
	Scotch or bourbon (1.5 oz.)	105	10.5	*Summary:* Some cocktails are "more expensive" than others.
	Bloody Mary (5 oz.)	116	11.6	
	Beer (12 oz.)	146	14.6	
	Light beer (12 oz.)	100	10	
	Martini (2.5 oz.)	156	15.6	
	Gin and Tonic, or Screwdriver (7.5 oz.)	174	17.4	
	▶ Mai Tai (4.5 oz.)	310	31	
Appetizers	Rice cakes (each)	35	3.5	*Summary:*
	Mini pretzels (20)	110	11	Choose your snacks carefully. ▶ Not all snacks are created equal.
	Potato chips (per ounce)	152	15.2	▶ Dry roasted nuts are still high calorie.
	Low fat potato chips (with Olestra)	75	7.5	▶ Trail mix sounds healthy, but check the calories carefully.
	Oriental rice mix (per ounce)	143	14.3	
	Cashews (per ounce)	160	16	
	Sunflower seeds (1 cup in the shell)	262	26.2	
	▶ Trail mix (per cup. Calories vary with composition)	693	69.3	
	Pistachios (per cup)	713	71.3	
	Peanuts (per cup)	828	82.8	
	▶ Mixed nuts, oil roasted (per cup)	886	88.6	
	▶ Mixed nuts, dry roasted (per cup)	814	81.4	

	Food	Calories	Year-Pounds (Approximate)	Simple Numbers to Remember and Points of Note
Main Courses	*Fish*			
	Broiled	70	7	*Summary:*
	Creole	158	15.8	▶ Fish is "what you do with it."
				▶ Watch "the skin" on poultry.
	Breaded	290	29	▶ All cuts of beef are not the same.
				▶ Lean ground turkey is a "bargain."
	▶ Almandine	347	34.7	
	Chicken			
	Breast broiled *without* skin	142	14.2	
	Breast broiled *with* skin	193	19.3	
	Breast fried *without* skin	161	16.1	
	Breast fried *with* skin	218	21.8	
	Pork (per 3 oz. Small!)			
	Tenderloin	141	14.1	
	Spareribs	337	33.7	
	Lamb chop (each)	255	25.5	
	Beef (per 3 oz. Small again!)			
	Porterhouse	173	17.3	
	Sirloin	280	28	
	Corned beef or brisket	315	31.5	
	Short ribs	357	35.7	
	▶ Tenderloin	530	53	
	Veal			
	Chop (lean only)	80	8	
	Veal parmigiana	267	26.7	
	▶ Veal cutlet (fried)	760	76	
	Meat loaf			
	▶ Turkey	110	11	
	▶ Beef	438	43.8	
	Pasta			
	Spaghetti marinara	185	18.5	
	Spaghetti with meat sauce	255	25.5	
	▶ Spaghetti with sausage	658	65.8	
	▶ Macaroni and cheese	430	43	

	Food	Calories	Year-Pounds (Approximate)	Simple Numbers to Remember and Points of Note
Vegetables and Potatoes	Cabbage	10	1	
				Summary:
(per serving)	Broccoli, asparagus, beets	24	2.4	Most veggies are a "bargain." ▶Not all beans are "beans."
	Carrots	31	3.1	▶Some beans are starch, right up there with pasta and potatoes.
	▶Artichoke	53	5.3	▶As with poultry, watch the skin on potatoes.
	▶Green beans	22	2.2	
	▶Pinto beans per cup	235	23.5	
	Potato			
	▶Baked with skin, no butter, etc.	220	22	
	▶Baked without skin, no butter, etc.	145	14.5	
	With butter add ...	36/Tbsp.	3.6	
	With sour cream add ...	30	3	
	With nonfat sour cream add ...	10	1	
	Au gratin	300	30	
	▶French fried	520	52	
	Sweet potato plain, fresh	180	18	
	Sweet potato (canned)	212	21.2	
	Rice plain, per cup	205	20.5	
Desserts	*Fruit*			*Summary:*
	Peach	37	3.7	Fresh fruit is generally a "bargain." ▶Dried fruit is another story.
	Apple	81	8.1	
	Pear	98	9.8	Occasional "to die for" desserts are fun, but compare and choose wisely.
	Banana	105	10.5	
	Blueberries per cup	82	8.2	
	Frozen, sweetened	187	18.7	
	Canned, in heavy syrup	224	22.4	
	Grapes per cup	58	5.8	
	▶Raisins (a.k.a. dried grapes) per ⅔ cup	300	30	

Food	Calories	Year-Pounds (Approximate)	Simple Numbers to Remember and Points of Note
Pies and cakes (per slice)			
Apple, peach, or cherry pie	302	30.2	
▶ Pecan pie	500	50	
Angel food cake	137	13.7	
Chocolate cake with icing	367	36.7	
▶ A national cheese cake restaurant's carrot cake			Remember: 120 extra calories a day is 12 pounds a year
(<u>per slice</u>)	1560	156	
Pudding			
Tapioca pudding	111	11.1	
Chocolate or rice pudding	192	19.2	
▶ Crème brulée	982	98.2	
Ice Cream, etc. (per ½ cup. Not much!)			
Light ice cream	120	12	
Sorbet	120	12	
▶ Full fat ice cream	270	27	

RECIPES (SORT OF)— FOOD FOR THOUGHT

Many books on dieting and weight loss have page upon page of low fat, low calorie recipes. Many of these recipes may not suit your taste. Perhaps you keep *your* favorite recipes stuffed into a binder in a kitchen drawer. Rather than give you yet more recipes to store, I want to show you how to change your favorites to help shed extra ounces. You don't need a new cookbook, unless you want to buy a new one that really interests you. You can simply apply a few changes to your favorite meals. Rather than deal with the actual recipes though, I think it more efficient to deal with principles and the exchange of ingredients. Food for thought.

Recall that fat contains over twice the calories—twice the *year-pounds*—of carbohydrates and protein. The former is nine calories per gram; the latter, four calories per gram. Of course, you have never seen a calorie, or picked up a gram. Therefore, for the sake of simplification, we will stick with calories converted to *year-pounds*. A *year-pound* is the extra weight attributed to eating an item daily for a year, in excess of usual caloric intake. Fat contains 4086 calories per pound, or 408.6 *year-pounds*. Carbohydrates and protein contain 1816 calories per pound, or 181.6 *year-pounds*.

Recall that eating larger portions of lower calorie items gets you nothing. With this in mind, let's work on a few recipes and principles to illustrate how to save four ounces a week, and then some. This will be in addition to any commitment you can make to reduce portion size. Combining reduced calories in an item with reduced portion size is additive. Throw in a little exercise and you are on your way.

The six basic principles are simple. Short and sweet so to speak.

▶ Replace fat items with low fat or nonfat items whenever possible.

▶ Use as little fat or oil as possible.

▶ Replace beef with lean turkey breast or lean pork loin where possible.

▶ Use the highest comfortable proportion of vegetables to meat or poultry in dishes such as stir-fries, stews, casseroles, etc.

▶ When baking, exchange one-third to one-half of the oil with applesauce or mashed ripe banana.

▶ Use egg substitute or egg whites instead of whole eggs, adding about two egg whites per one egg. (One egg = 75 cal. One egg white = 16 cal. One half cup typical egg substitute = 30 cal.)

And of course: Eat less.

Some recipes

Below are the ingredients in a few favorite recipes. Notice how changing ingredients affects weight loss. Take a few minutes to study these ingredients, and then experiment on your own. Adjust your favorite recipes, but realize not all recipes are adaptable to change. *There is no low fat crème bruleé.* Sometimes color or consistency will vary, even if the taste is the same. You will need to decide if this matters. These are examples to show the general principle of food modification. Do your own thing. Experiment. I think you will be amazed how many calories you can cut out, and actually have fun looking for those extra few calories to shed. Find the loose change under the sofa cushions.

▶ *Remember: You only need to shave eight hundred and forty calories a week to meet your goal of a quarter pound a week, so pay particular attention to the third column.* ◀

Original Recipe	Altered Recipe	Calories and *year-pounds* saved (*per recipe not per serving*)
Baked Manicotti 1	**Baked Manicotti 2**	-960 calories *96 year-pounds*
1 package manicotti	1 package manicotti	
8 oz. ricotta cheese ▶	8 oz. low fat ricotta cheese	
8 oz. mozzarella cheese ▶	8 oz. low fat mozzarella cheese	
32 oz. jar marinara sauce	32 oz. jar marinara sauce	
Quiche Lorraine 1	**Quiche Lorraine 2**	-987 calories *98.7 year-pounds*
9-inch pie shell (*960 calories*)	9-inch pie shell	
2 cups half & half ▶	2 cups nonfat half & half	
3 eggs ▶	4 egg whites plus 1 whole egg	
½ tsp. salt	½ tsp. salt	
½ tsp. pepperr	½ tsp. pepper	
½ tsp. nutmeg	½ tsp. nutmeg	
¼ pound bacon ▶	¼ pound ham or turkey bacon	
½ cup Swiss cheese ▶	½ cup fat free Swiss cheese	
Beef Meatloaf	**Turkey Meatloaf**	-583 calories *58.3 year-pounds*
1 pound ground beef ▶	1 pound ground turkey (white meat)	
2 eggs ▶	4 egg whites	
¼ cup ketchup	¼ cup ketchup	
1 sm. chopped onion	1 sm. chopped onion	
1 ½–2 cups oatmeal	1 ½–2 cups oatmeal	
½ cup milk ▶	½ cup nonfat milk	
½ tsp. parsley flakes	½ tsp. parsley flakes	
¼ tsp. pepper	¼ tsp. pepper	

Original Recipe	Altered Recipe	Calories and *year-pounds* saved (*per recipe not per serving*)
Hungarian Mushroom Soup 1	**Hungarian Mushroom Soup 2**	-474 calories *47.4 year-pounds*
4 Tbsp. butter ▶	4 Tbsp. low fat butter substitute	
2 cups chicken broth ▶	2 cups low fat chicken broth	
1 cup milk ▶	1 cup nonfat milk	
½ cup sour cream ▶	½ cup nonfat sour cream	
1 pound mushrooms	1 pound mushrooms	
1 Tbsp. paprika	1 Tbsp. paprika	
1 Tbsp. soy sauce	1 Tbsp. soy sauce	
3 Tbsp. flour	3 Tbsp. flour	
2 tsp. lemon juice	2 tsp. lemon juice	
¼ cup parsley	¼ cup parsley	
Chocolate Cake & Frosting 1	**Chocolate Cake & Frosting 2**	-605 calories *60.5 year-pounds*
Cake	*Cake*	
2 cups sugar	2 cups sugar	
1 ¾ cups flour	1 ¾ cups flour	
¾ cup cocoa	¾ cup cocoa	
1 ½ tsp. baking soda	1 ½ tsp. baking soda	
1 ½ tsp. baking powder	1 ½ tsp. baking powder	
1 tsp. salt	1 tsp. salt	
2 eggs ▶	½ cup egg substitute	
1 cup milk ▶	1 cup nonfat milk	
½ cup vegetable oil ▶	¼ cup vegetable oil plus ¼ cup applesauce	
2 tsp. vanilla	2 tsp. vanilla	
Frosting	*Frosting*	
½ cup butter	½ cup butter (no change)	
⅔ cup cocoa	⅔ cup cocoa	
3 cups powdered sugar	3 cups powdered sugar	
⅓ cup milk ▶	⅓ cup nonfat milk	
1 tsp. vanilla	1 tsp. vanilla	

Stretchable Vegetables

▶**You need to read this.**

My wife and daughter, masters at shaving calories off recipes, taught me this principle. Vegetables are low calorie and very tasty if used correctly. Yes, your mother was right when she said, "Eat your vegetables." *A wonderful trick is to use vegetables to stretch high calorie items like cheese to lower the calories per serving.*

Let me give you an example. Take the manicotti recipe. Add a package of thawed frozen spinach to the cheese mixture. The spinach adds a delicious flavor and dilutes the cheese per serving, thereby reducing the calories and *year-pounds.*

Similarly, you can stretch the calories of the quiche by adding spinach, sautéed red peppers, and onions. Be sure to sauté the vegetables in a *minimal* amount of oil or low fat butter substitute. I think you'll find these additions not only save calories, but also add flavor. Use any vegetable you'd like; you're not limited to spinach. Perhaps consider a crustless quiche, a frittata, and save nine hundred and sixty extra calories. Experiment. Enjoy.

NOTES

1. Leah Hoffmann and Lacey Rose, "What 10 diet plans cost," 12 April 2005. http://moneycentral.msn.com.

2. Alain J. Nordmann Abigail Nordmann, Matthias Briel, et al., "Effects of low-carbohydrate vs. low-fat diets on weight loss and cardiovascular risk factors: a meta-analysis of randomized controlled trials," *Archives of Internal Medicine* (2006), 166:285–293.

3. AM Wolf and GA Colditz, "Current estimates of the economic cost of obesity in the United States," *Obesity Research* (1998), 6:97–106.

4. "U.S. obesity cost: $96.7 B," 3 June 2005. http://www.redherring.com.

5. "Overweight", 6 October 2006. http://www.cdc.gov/nchs/fastats/overwt.htm.

6. "U.S. obesity cost: $96.7 B," 3 June 2005. http://www.redherring.com.

7. John F. Banzhaf, "HHS OKs penalizing obese for health insurance," http://banzhaf.net/docs/fatrates.

8. "Obesity weighs heavily on airlines," February 2005. http://www.popsci.com.

9. Leah Hoffmann and Lacey Rose, 12 April 2005.

10. Leah Hoffmann and Lacey Rose, 12 April 2005.

11. Michael L. Dansinger, MD, Joi Augustin Gleason, MS, RD, John L. Griffith, PhD, Harry P. Selker, MD, MSPH, Ernst J. Schaefer, MD, "Comparison of the Atkins, Ornish, Weight Watchers, and Zone diets for weight loss and heart disease risk reduction," *The Journal of the American Medical Association* (2005), 293:43–53.

12. Thomas A. Wadden, PhD, Robert L. Berkowitz, MD, Leslie G. Womble, PhD, et al., "Randomized trial of lifestyle modification and pharmacotherapy for obesity," *The New England Journal of Medicine* (2005), 353:2111–2120.

13. Dansinger 43.

14. Dansinger 43.

15. Dena M. Bravata, MD, MS, Lisa Sanders, MD, Jane Huang, MD, et al., "Efficacy and safety of low-carbohydrate diets," *The Journal of the American Medical Association* (2003), 289:1837–1850.

978-0-595-39963-5
0-595-39963-0

Printed in the United States
78903LV00007B/331